Toward A National Health Care Survey

A Data System for the 21st Century

Gooloo S. Wunderlich, *Editor*

Panel on the National Health Care Survey
Edward B. Perrin and William C. Richardson, *Cochairs*

Committee on National Statistics
Commission on Behavioral and Social Sciences and Education
National Research Council

Division of Health Care Services
Institute of Medicine

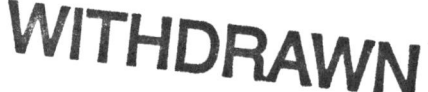

National Academy Press
Washington, D.C. 1992

NOTICE: The project that is the subject of this report was approved by the Governing Board of the National Research Council, whose members are drawn from the councils of the National Academy of Sciences, the National Academy of Engineering, and the Institute of Medicine. The members of the committee responsible for the report were chosen for their special competences and with regard for appropriate balance.

This report has been reviewed by a group other than the authors according to procedures approved by a Report Review Committee consisting of members of the National Academy of Sciences, the National Academy of Engineering, and the Institute of Medicine.

The National Academy of Sciences is a private, nonprofit, self-perpetuating society of distinguished scholars engaged in scientific and engineering research, dedicated to the furtherance of science and technology and to their use for the general welfare. Upon the authority of the charter granted to it by the Congress in 1863, the Academy has a mandate that requires it to advise the federal government on scientific and technical matters. Dr. Frank Press is president of the National Academy of Sciences.

The National Academy of Engineering was established in 1964, under the charter of the National Academy of Sciences, as a parallel organization of outstanding engineers. It is autonomous in its administration and in the selection of its members, sharing with the National Academy of Sciences the responsibility for advising the federal government. The National Academy of Engineering also sponsors engineering programs aimed at meeting national needs, encourages education and research, and recognizes the superior achievements of engineers. Dr. Robert M. White is president of the National Academy of Engineering.

The Institute of Medicine was established in 1970 by the National Academy of Sciences to secure the services of eminent members of appropriate professions in the examination of policy matters pertaining to the health of the public. The Institute acts under the responsibility given to the National Academy of Sciences by its congressional charter to be an adviser to the federal government and, upon its own initiative, to identify issues of medical care, research, and education. Dr. Kenneth I. Shine is president of the Institute of Medicine.

The National Research Council was organized by the National Academy of Sciences in 1916 to associate the broad community of science and technology with the Academy's purposes of furthering knowledge and advising the federal government. Functioning in accordance with general policies determined by the Academy, the Council has become the principal operating agency of both the National Academy of Sciences and the National Academy of Engineering in providing services to the government, the public, and the scientific and engineering communities. The Council is administered jointly by both Academies and the Institute of Medicine. Dr. Frank Press and Dr. Robert M. White are chairman and vice chairman, respectively, of the National Research Council.

The project that is the subject of this report was supported by funds from the National Center for Health Statistics, U.S. Department of Health and Human Services (Contract No. 200-89-7020).

Library of Congress Catalog Card No. 92-80092
International Standard Book Number 0-309-04692-0

Additional copies of this report are available from:

National Academy Press
2101 Constitution Avenue, NW
Washington, DC 20418

S551

Printed in the United States of America

PANEL ON THE NATIONAL HEALTH CARE SURVEY

EDWARD B. PERRIN (*Cochair*), School of Public Health and Community Medicine, University of Washington
WILLIAM C. RICHARDSON (*Cochair*), President, Johns Hopkins University
LINDA AIKEN, Department of Sociology, University of Pennsylvania
ROBERT L. BLACK, Private Pediatric Practice, Monterey, California
JOHN W. COLLOTON,[*] The University of Iowa Hospitals and Clinics
JOHN COOMBS, Statistics Canada, Ottawa, Ontario
SUZANNE W. FLETCHER, Annals of Internal Medicine, Philadelphia, Pennsylvania
FLOYD J. FOWLER, Center for Survey Research, University of Massachusetts
DANIEL G. HORVITZ, Research Triangle Institute, Research Triangle Park, North Carolina
WILLIAM KALSBEEK, Department of Biostatistics, University of North Carolina
GRAHAM KALTON,[**] Survey Research Center, Institute for Social Research, University of Michigan
SIDNEY KATZ, School of Medicine and Public Health, Columbia University
DAVID MECHANIC, Institute for Health, Health Care Policy, and Aging Research, Rutgers University
JOSEPH NEWHOUSE, Division of Health Policy Research and Education, Harvard University
ADRIAN M. OSTFELD, Department of Epidemiology and Public Health, Yale University School of Medicine

GOOLOO S. WUNDERLICH, *Study Director*
ANU PEMMARAZU, *Senior Project Assistant*

---

[*]Served until May 1991
[**]As of January 1992, senior statistician and vice president, Westat, Inc.

COMMITTEE ON NATIONAL STATISTICS
1991-1992

BURTON H. SINGER (*Chair*), Department of Epidemiology and Public Health, Yale University

NORMAN M. BRADBURN, National Opinion Research Center, University of Chicago

MARTIN H. DAVID, Department of Economics, University of Wisconsin

ANGUS S. DEATON, Woodrow Wilson School of Public and International Affairs, Princeton University

NOREEN GOLDMAN, Office of Population Research, Princeton University

LOUIS GORDON, Department of Mathematics, University of Southern California

JOEL B. GREENHOUSE, Department of Statistics, Carnegie Mellon University

ROBERT M. HAUSER, Department of Sociology, University of Wisconsin

GRAHAM KALTON,* Survey Research Center, Institute for Social Research, University of Michigan

WILLIAM A. MORRILL, Mathtech, Inc., Princeton, New Jersey

DOROTHY P. RICE, Department of Social and Behavioral Sciences, School of Nursing, University of California, San Francisco

JOHN E. ROLPH, The RAND Corporation, Santa Monica, California

DONALD B. RUBIN, Department of Statistics, Harvard University

MIRON L. STRAF, *Director*
SUSANNA MCFARLAND, *Administrative Assistant*

---

*As of January 1992, Westat, Inc.

INSTITUTE OF MEDICINE

Board on Health Care Services

WALTER J. MCNERNEY (*Chair*), J.L. Kellog Graduate School of Management, Northwestern University
BEN D. BARKER, School of Dentistry, University of North Carolina
LONNIE R. BRISTOW, San Pablo, California
EDWARD J. CONNERS, Mercy Health Services, Farmington Hills, Michigan
DON E. DETMER, Health Sciences Center, University of Virginia
CHARLES C. EDWARDS, Scripps Clinic & Research Foundation, La Jolla, California
PAUL F. GRINER, University of Rochester Medical Center, Strong Memorial Hospital, Rochester, New York
CLARK C. HAVIGHURST, Duke University School of Law
SIDNEY KATZ, School of Medicine and Public Health, Columbia University
JOSEPH P. NEWHOUSE, Division of Health Policy Research and Education, Harvard University
ROBERT PATRICELLI, Value Health, Inc., Avon, Connecticut
EDWARD B. PERRIN, School of Public Health and Community Medicine, University of Washington
RICHARD J. REITEMEIER, Phoenix Alliance, St. Paul, Minnesota
GAIL L. WARDEN, Henry Ford Health Care Corporation, Detroit, Michigan

KARL D. YORDY, *Division Director*
KATHLEEN N. LOHR, *Deputy Director*
H. DONALD TILLER, *Administrative Assistant*

Acknowledgments

The Panel on the National Health Care Survey gratefully acknowledges the contributions of the many individuals who participated and gave generously of their time and knowledge to this study.

Support for the study was provided by the National Center for Health Statistics (NCHS) of the U.S. Department of Health and Human Services. The NCHS staff was very helpful in providing information about the center's health care surveys and in responding to numerous inquiries and requests throughout the study. We particularly wish to thank W. Edward Bacon, director of the Division of Health Care Statistics and the NCHS project officer, for his assistance throughout our deliberations. In addition, we would like to acknowledge the many federal and nonfederal government officials and those from the research community who participated in the survey of users conducted by the panel. Finally, thoughtful and helpful comments on our report were received from the many reviewers within the National Research Council, including members of the Committee on National Statistics, the Commission on Behavioral and Social Sciences and Education, the Institute of Medicine, and other external experts.

We acknowledge with gratitude the contributions of staff. The panel is especially grateful for the guidance and the unstinting efforts of the study director, Gooloo S. Wunderlich, who had primary responsibility for organizing the deliberations of the panel and preparing the draft of the final report, tasks that she accomplished with considerable skill and good humor.

In addition, we would like to thank Kathleen N. Lohr, Division of Health Care Services, Institute of Medicine, who prepared much of the material for Chapter 2 of the report. Early in the project, Ruth S. Hanft, professor in the Department of Health Services Management and Policy at the George Washington University, prepared a background paper for the panel on issues of health care delivery and the associated data needs. We also acknowledge the efforts of project consultants Michael Cohen, in preparation of discussion drafts on statistical issues associated with the survey design, and Earl Pollack, especially for assistance in the early stages of the study and in the survey of users. Christine McShane, editor for the Commission on Behavioral and Social Sciences and Education, provided highly professional editorial advice on the report. The support and guidance of Karl D. Yordy, Division of Health Care Services, Institute of Medicine, as well as his assistance in the review and revision of the report, deserve special mention. The study would not have been possible without the dedicated efforts of Anu Pemmarazu, senior project assistant, in participating in the survey of users, preparing summary reports and synthesizing the findings for panel meetings, managing logistics for the large number of panel meetings, and competently handling the various drafts of the report.

Finally, we would like to thank the members of the panel for their generous contribution of time and expert knowledge to the deliberations and the preparation of this report.

Edward B. Perrin, *Cochair*
William C. Richardson, *Cochair*
Panel on the National Health Care Survey

Contents

EXECUTIVE SUMMARY 1
    Findings and Conclusions, 3
    Recommendations, 10

1   INTRODUCTION 15
    Panel's Charge and Its Approach, 16
    Organization of the Report, 18

2   DATA NEEDS FOR A CHANGING HEALTH CARE
    DELIVERY SYSTEM 19
    Three Critical Issues in Health Care, 20
    Health Care Reform, 28
    Other Factors Influencing Health Care Policy
       and Data Needs, 29
    Users of Health Care Data, 37
    Implications for Data Sources and Systems, 38

3   REVIEW OF THE NCHS PLAN FOR THE NATIONAL
    HEALTH CARE SURVEY 41
    Overview, 41
    Periodicity, 43
    Scope and Coverage, 46

Data Collected, 49
Design Features, 52
Conclusion, 60

4 DESIGN FOR A NATIONAL HEALTH CARE
   DATA SYSTEM 62
   Statement of Objectives, 63
   Design Considerations, 64
   A Framework for a National Health Care
     Data System, 65
   Potential Benefits of the Proposed Design
     Framework, 78
   Implementation Strategy, 80

5 COORDINATION AND RESOURCE CONSIDERATIONS 83
   Advisory Structure for the National Health
     Care Data System, 83
   Improving Departmental Coordination, 86
   Enhancing the Center's Analytic Capability, 88
   Resource Requirements, 89

APPENDICES
   A NCHS Plan for a National Health Care Survey, 93
   B Survey of Users of National Health Care Statistics, 111
   C Federal Health Data Sources, 125
   D Statutory Authorities, 151
   E Acronyms, 167
   F Biographical Sketches, 169

SOURCES AND REFERENCES 175

Toward A National Health Care Survey

Executive Summary

The nation's health care system has changed dramatically during the past two decades. Health policy makers and researchers have a compelling need for more and better data on a number of issues if they are to understand and solve the current health care problems facing the nation. The national health statistical systems have not kept pace with the changing and increasing demand for information that this rapidly evolving health care delivery environment has generated. The gaps in information on a wide array of issues concerning health are growing. The current national data systems are becoming outdated. They do not provide the information needed to allow researchers and policy makers to assess adequately the effect of changes in the financing, organization, and delivery of health care, or the impact of other social and economic trends, on the appropriateness, quality, costs, and outcomes of care.

Recognizing that existing national data systems need to be more responsive to the changes occurring in the health care system, the National Center for Health Statistics (NCHS) in the U.S. Public Health Service is developing a plan for restructuring its existing surveys of health care providers and service settings[1] into what it has chosen to call an integrated National Health Care Survey. Under its plan the National Health Care

---

[1] The surveys are the National Hospital Discharge Survey, the National Ambulatory Medical Care Survey, The National Nursing Home Survey, and the National Master Facility Inventory.

Survey will build on the existing provider surveys, which will be merged and expanded over time and geographically linked with the National Health Interview Survey (NHIS). The aim of this proposed new survey is to provide a more complete and useful picture than now exists of the provision of medical care in the United States. The main features of the NCHS plan are:

- To conduct the survey on an annual basis;
- To expand the coverage of types of health care providers and health service settings to include hospital emergency and outpatient departments, ambulatory surgery centers, home health agencies, and hospices;
- To revise the sample design using a three-stage cluster design in which a subset of the primary sample of the NHIS will be used to select the sample for the independently designed provider-based surveys; and
- To develop a capability to conduct follow-up studies to examine issues related to outcome and subsequent medical care.

NCHS requested that the National Academy of Sciences and the Institute of Medicine convene a panel of experts to evaluate their plans for the National Health Care Survey. The panel was asked to undertake two major tasks in this evaluation:

(1) Identify the principal current and future needs for health care data by public and private policy makers, health care providers, health service researchers, and others and

(2) Determine the extent to which the proposed survey can meet identified needs for data given the statistical aspects of the proposed survey, such as sample design, sample size, data collection methods, and data sets.

This report responds to this request. It reviews the main features of the proposed survey from two perspectives: the extent to which the survey would enable NCHS to meet the changing data needs associated with the health care policy issues identified by the panel, and the technical features of the plan in its current stage of development. It goes beyond a simple review of NCHS plans, however, to suggest a broader strategy for the surveys that the panel believes will more nearly meet the needs of the health care system.

The panel's major findings and conclusions based on this review and its deliberations are summarized below, followed by the text of its recommendations.

FINDINGS AND CONCLUSIONS

In reviewing the key features of, and developments in, health care and the array of national health data sources available, it became clear to the panel that, although there is an abundance of data collection activities in this nation, they often are uncoordinated and are sometimes duplicative. Moreover, they do not provide the full range of statistical information needed to monitor and evaluate changes in the availability, financing, and quality of health care in order to meet today's challenges, let alone the challenges of the next century.

It also became clear to the panel that no single survey is likely ever to meet all the criteria, address all the technical problems, or meet all users' needs for data. In order to be able to meet future demands for information, a coordinated and integrated system of health care data collection activities involving several organizational entities is required. Collectively such a data system should be flexible enough to adapt to the changes in the health care system as they occur and to meet special needs on an ad hoc basis.

NCHS Plan for a National Health Care Survey

The panel commends NCHS for taking the first steps in restructuring and expanding the existing health provider surveys to enhance the amount and kind of information available about health care events. The panel endorses the concept of a National Health Care Survey integrated with the National Health Interview Survey to monitor the nation's health, illness, and disability; the use of and costs of care by incident and episode; and the outcomes and cost-effectiveness of the services provided. Such monitoring and evaluation should broadly examine both general and mental health and related disabilities.

The panel has reviewed the main features of the survey as proposed in the NCHS plan. In its judgment the plan in its present stage of development does not provide the capacity to address important questions about the interrelationships between the health status of individuals and the patterns and cost of health care services they receive from a broad range of health care providers and service settings over time. Therefore the panel believes that it is important for it to provide guidance that would redirect the planning process. The timing is also opportune, since NCHS is currently in the midst of planning the 1995 redesign of NHIS, which will affect NHIS data collection for several years. NCHS should take into consideration the panel's recommendations relating to their plans for the proposed National Health Care Survey in reaching final decisions on the NHIS redesign. The panel's major findings and conclusions follow:

- The panel supports the annual data collection schedule planned by NCHS, but it is concerned about further reducing the already small sample sizes to offset increased costs. Such action will further aggravate the existing problems of producing estimates for subpopulations, for rare diseases and diagnoses, and for subnational levels. NCHS proposes to address that problem by aggregating data over more than a year. Such multiyear aggregation of data may be less appropriate for characteristics that are not stable across years. It will also affect the timeliness of data production and analysis. Moreover, the panel seriously doubts the possibility of producing small-area estimates even with the proposed aggregation of data over multiple years.

- The panel endorses the center's plan to extend coverage of the health care provider surveys to include additional health care settings that have emerged in recent years. However, further extensions are needed to include a fuller range of providers than currently planned—both physicians and nonphysicians. Examples of these would include dentists, psychologists, occupational therapists, pharmacists, podiatrists, chiropractors, nurses, nurse practitioners, physician assistants, nurse midwives, and optometrists, all of whom deliver some form of health care. The panel also finds the exclusion of federal hospitals and long-term care hospitals a serious deficiency in the present plan.

- Although the panel is in general agreement with the topics currently included in the health care provider surveys, it finds the content inadequate to meet the data needs for the current and future health care policy issues. Some of the key issues not addressed in the center's plan are summarized below:

    — Information on longitudinal dimensions of care is of critical importance to assess the effects of treatment, but current data sets do not permit data aggregation to depict meaningful patterns of care over time. Person-based data are needed on health care received by individuals over time and over the entire progression of an episode of illness.

    — The cost of care is one of the most, if not the most, important health policy issues confronting the nation today, yet hardly any information is collected by NCHS in the health care provider surveys on payers or health care costs and expenditures, including the component paid by insurance. Section 306 of the Public Health Service Act, which provides the statutory mandate for NCHS, lists the specific areas in which statistics are to be collected. These mandated areas cover health resources, the utilization of health care, and health care costs and financing, including the trends in health care prices and costs, the sources of payments for health services, and federal, state, and local government expenditures for health care.

— Data on readmissions to hospitals and multiple visits to ambulatory care settings are not available because the information obtained is on discharges and visits in the provider surveys and not on persons.

— A major limitation, not only of NCHS surveys but of virtually all data sets about health care services, is the lack of detailed information on the tests and services performed during the various treatment events. The addition of such data from medical records or charts to the content of the survey is critical to research related to the appropriateness of care, the outcomes and efficacy of treatments, and the costs of treatment.

As stated earlier, a central feature of the center's plan is to link geographically the sample selection of the provider surveys with the sampling design of the NHIS by using a subsample of the NHIS primary sampling units to select the samples for the independently designed provider surveys. NCHS has identified several potential advantages of the revised design:

- The panel concludes that there may be some practical advantages to having the provider surveys and the NHIS conducted in the same primary sampling units (PSUs). There may be efficiencies in sharing data collection staff, although the real benefits cannot be assessed until the actual strategies for data collection are fully in place. Furthermore, the assumed cost saving of having the health care providers geographically clustered needs to be demonstrated. The trade-off between reduced costs through use of a clustered provider sample and the impact of this design on the efficiency of the sample also needs to be examined in greater detail.

- NCHS has given considerable thought to the concept of an integrated National Health Care Survey and has presented arguments that its plan implies integration. Although the panel supports the use of the NHIS PSUs as an important first step, it emphasizes that simply conducting the provider surveys in the NHIS PSUs does not by itself result in a meaningfully integrated survey.

- The panel is skeptical about the assumptions of increased analytic utility resulting from geographic linkage, and it doubts there is benefit in defining the PSUs in terms of health service areas. There are several problems associated with the definition of health service areas across a range of health services and health care providers that need to be researched before the utility of this kind of analysis can be assessed. The health service area concept, of course, can be used in analyses of NCHS survey data without using the concept to define PSUs.

- The NCHS plan for a National Health Care Survey includes development of the capability to conduct routine and specialized patient follow-up studies of the sample event—visit, discharge or admission—to obtain information beyond what is available in provider records. Although the follow-up design described by NCHS potentially adds somewhat to the value of the data currently being collected, in the panel's judgment the key issue is the appropriateness of an event-based sample for follow-up studies. *A major limitation of the National Health Care Survey as presently designed is that all the provider surveys begin with a sample of events and not with a sample of persons.* This is not an efficient design for producing person-based statistics. Many health conditions produce multiple visits to an ambulatory care setting; NCHS needs to determine the extent of the confounding problem resulting from the use of an event-based survey. There are also statistical problems that need to be resolved, arising from the fact that an individual's chance of selection in the sample depends on the number of health care events he or she had for the condition.

In conclusion, the panel endorses the primary objective of the planned survey "to produce annual data on the use of health care and the outcomes of care for the major sectors of the health care delivery system. These data will describe the patient population, medical care provided, financing, and provider characteristics." The panel is concerned, however, that, as currently designed, the survey appears to be limited mostly to modest modifications and expansions in coverage and content of the existing health care provider surveys with minimal, if any, true integration of design or data. If the center's objective is to move in the direction of an integrated survey design to provide comprehensive health care data that are urgently needed, especially on the key dimensions of access, expenditures, illness episodes, and outcomes, in the opinion of the panel, it must move beyond the event-based sampling procedures that are proposed in its plan.

Design Framework for a National Health Care Data System

In reviewing the features of the NCHS plan, the panel concludes that, even taking the panel's recommendations for changes and improvements in the current plan into account, the center's vision for a National Health Care Survey falls short of meeting anticipated information needs for the critical years ahead and into the next century. Long-term strategy requires consideration of further, more fundamental restructuring of the surveys to produce a plan that is flexible enough to adapt to changes and to new and rapidly emerging needs for health care data. Such a strategy requires a more integrated and a more visionary course of action than currently set forth by NCHS. As stated at the outset, no one survey can meet all the requirements and provide answers to all the important health care questions, but considerably more can be done than has been proposed by NCHS thus far.

The panel believes that there is need to develop an integrated data system with linkage capability at the individual level that includes a variety of approaches, including surveys of specific types of health care providers and health care settings, follow-up of individuals seen for specific conditions by specific types of providers in specific settings, longitudinal surveys of the household and nursing home populations, and possibly surveys of episodes of illness. In addition, there is need for improved collaboration, coordination, and integration of health care data collected by NCHS and by other agencies of the U.S. Department of Health and Human Services.

The panel therefore recommends a more ambitious course of action that will provide the basis for a flexible, long-term data collection strategy, one that encompasses most of the features of the present NCHS plan, but that calls for a significant long-term expansion in the breadth and depth of information to be gathered through a truly integrated National Health Care Data System.

This report presents the panel's strategy for achieving these objectives, not so much as a specific design but as a design framework for an integrated National Health Care Data System within which a variety of survey approaches linked to the NHIS can be developed, and from which a broad range of health-related information needs can be met. This approach would provide not only new data, but also a basis for linkage of data on a population-based sample of individuals with data on their health care providers. The panel believes that, taken as a totality, its recommended course of action represents the appropriate and preferred direction for the National Health Care Data System.

The panel's proposed design framework has four key elements:

(1) Changing the origin of the provider samples from listings of providers and service settings developed and maintained by NCHS to identification of providers and service settings by respondents to the NHIS (at least for those health care providers not currently included in the provider inventories maintained by NCHS). This NHIS-based approach offers rapid identification of emerging health care providers and service settings, which is just not possible with

the current approach of developing and maintaining national inventories for given types of providers to serve as sampling frames.

(2) Sampling from the NHIS respondents to gather longitudinal person-based data on the health status and health care sought and received by individuals, including what services were provided by which providers, along with the associated costs and expenditures.

(3) Modifying the sampling design of the National Nursing Home Survey (NNHS) to collect longitudinal data from the institutionalized population on health care utilization from providers other than the nursing home.

(4) Generating a sample of episodes of illness from respondents to the NHIS and the NNHS. These respondents with an episode of illness will be followed over a period of time to collect data from both the respondents and their health care providers on the process of health care, the utilization of providers, and costs and expenditures associated with the episode.

The panel recognizes that, despite its many potential benefits, adoption of the recommended design framework raises several important issues on various aspects that would require careful examination and resolution as to feasibility and costs prior to making final decisions on the details of the design. Many of the issues identified are related to some of the screening and patient follow-up procedures. Perhaps the most important pertain to the ability: (1) to identify visits to specific providers, (2) to obtain information making possible contact with identified providers, (3) to obtain permission from patients to contact the providers they have identified and to access their records, and then (4) to successfully enroll the providers and the patients in the survey.

Although the concept of the episodes of illness as a unit of analysis is attractive and such data would prove to be a very valuable analytical database, especially for medical effectiveness research, the panel recognizes that experience with its application is limited and problematic, especially as it applies to chronic illness episodes. Developing the capability to generate data on episodes of various types of illness raises important and complex methodological issues associated with the definition, classification, and measurement that should be researched by NCHS in collaboration with the Agency for Health Care Policy and Research in a systematic manner.

The panel concludes that NCHS should establish a research agenda to examine the issues on the various aspects of the proposed design framework prior to making final decisions on the specific details of the design.

EXECUTIVE SUMMARY 9

The panel outlines a phased multiyear strategy starting in 1992 for implementing its proposed data content, coverage, and design framework for a National Health Care Data System.

Coordination and Resource Considerations

In the course of the study the panel has noted several issues not directly addressed in its charge, some broadly related to the activities of NCHS and others that go beyond to the structural issues of collaboration and coordination of data gathering and analysis within the Department of Health and Human Services. The panel strongly believes that these broader issues must be addressed in the context of this report because the successful implementation of an integrated and effective National Health Care Data System will, to a large extent, depend on their resolution.

The panel believes that the concept and operations of the proposed National Health Care Data System should undergo external review by a panel of experts from outside the government. Furthermore, the panel has found that the internal analytical capabilities of NCHS, especially in its survey divisions, have been reduced in the past several years. This not only affects the timely analysis and interpretation of data collected, but also leads to the inability to anticipate important issues and to respond to them. The panel believes that, if not corrected, this deficiency will impair the ability of NCHS to implement the National Health Care Data System.

The panel further notes the fragmented state of the federal health statistics activities and concludes that the Department of Health and Human Services needs to undertake a major review of the vast array of its data collection activities related to health care with the objective of developing a comprehensive and coordinated plan for establishing an efficient and cost-effective structure and organization for health care statistics.

Finally, the panel emphasizes that without infusion of substantial new resources the course of action charted in this report cannot be accomplished, and the nation will continue to fall further behind in meeting its health care data needs. Health care data are of interest not only in terms of the general functions of NCHS, but more importantly in terms of specific use and interest in the establishment and evaluation of federal policy in health care. The panel considers the immediate implementation of its recommendations justified in view of the importance of health care information to the Congress and the executive branch in the establishment and evaluation of federal health care policy, as well as to the states and society as a whole as they cope with the significant changes in the organization and delivery of health care.

The panel recommends a considerably expanded data collection effort and a redesign strategy that will yield significantly more useful data than are currently available. An underfunded program cannot meet the needs of society effectively. In the final analysis, the commitment and institutional support of the secretary of the Department of Health and Human Services, the Office of Management and Budget, and the Congress are all essential to the successful implementation of a comprehensive integrated health care statistics strategy.

RECOMMENDATIONS

On the basis of its findings and conclusions the panel provides three categories of recommendations: (1) on the plan submitted by NCHS for review, (2) on the design framework for an integrated National Health Care Data System, and (3) on coordination, advice, and resource considerations. The text of the panel's recommendations, grouped according to these categories, follows, keyed to the chapter in which they appear in the body of the report.

RECOMMENDATIONS ON THE NCHS PLAN

Recommendation 3-1: The panel endorses the NCHS plan to conduct the provider surveys on an annual basis.

Recommendation 3-2: The panel recommends that NCHS extend its coverage of providers of health care to include a fuller range of health providers than currently planned—both physicians and nonphysicians, all of whom provide some form of health care. The panel further recommends that the universe for the hospital care component be extended to include long-term care hospitals and federal hospitals.

Recommendation 3-3: The panel recommends that NCHS put in place a mechanism for developing criteria and for setting data collection priorities across the full range of health care providers and service settings, and that this mechanism and process be dynamic and include periodic review and revisions of both the criteria and coverage as necessary.

Recommendation 3-4: The panel recommends that the National Health Care Survey include collection of *person-based* longitudinal information, expanding the data collected to include, but not be limited to, information on the health care received, costs and gross expenditures for health care, and outcomes.

Recommendation 3-5: The panel endorses the NCHS decision to use the primary sampling units from the National Health Interview Survey for the National Health Care Survey, to retain their existing definition at this time, and to continue the needed research in this area.

RECOMMENDATIONS FOR A DESIGN FRAMEWORK FOR THE NATIONAL HEALTH CARE DATA SYSTEM

Recommendation 4-1: The panel recommends that providers other than those currently covered—i.e., short-term hospitals, office-based physicians, and nursing homes—be surveyed using provider samples generated from the list of providers visited by respondents to the National Health Interview Survey as identified through the survey screening.

Recommendation 4-2: The panel recommends that NCHS examine the feasibility and utility of selecting its samples of short-term hospitals and office-based physicians from inventories of each of these types of providers visited by respondents to the National Health Interview Survey and identified through the survey screening.

Recommendation 4-3: The panel recommends that NCHS develop and implement, as a component of the National Health Care Data System, a continuous, longitudinal survey of health care utilization and expenditures, and their health care providers, using cohorts of individuals selected from among National Health Interview Survey respondents.

Recommendation 4-4: The panel recommends that NCHS develop and implement a survey capability to obtain longitudinal data for cohorts of residents of nursing homes, while institutionalized, on their use of and expenditures for health care received from providers other than the nursing home itself. NCHS should explore the possibility of obtaining this information for residents of other long-term institutions.

Continued

Recommendation 4-5: The panel recommends that NCHS undertake research in collaboration with the Agency for Health Care Policy and Research to examine the methodological issues of definitions and classifications and to determine the feasibility of using the National Health Interview Survey and the National Nursing Home Survey to generate a sample of episodes of illness; the sample should be followed longitudinally to collect data on the associated medical care use for the episode from both the sample of individuals and the health care providers.

Recommendation 4-6: The panel recommends that NCHS conduct research and develop procedures for data systems that enable linkage of health care outcomes to health care received and health care costs. The panel further urges NCHS to examine the feasibility of collecting health insurance claims files from both private and public insurers for individuals included in the samples from the National Health Interview Survey and the National Nursing Home Survey selected to study health care utilization and costs.

Recommendation 4-7: The panel recommends that NCHS take into serious consideration the recommendations in this report relating to the National Health Care Data System before reaching final decisions on the 1995 redesign of the National Health Interview Survey.

Recommendation 4-8: The panel recommends that NCHS establish a research agenda to determine the feasibility of its recommended course of action. If found feasible, the panel recommends that NCHS adopt the proposed design framework (with adjustments as warranted by the research) for a National Health Care Data System.

RECOMMENDATIONS RELATING TO COORDINATION AND RESOURCE CONSIDERATIONS

Recommendation 5-1: The panel recommends that a continuing external oversight group of health care professionals be established to monitor and advise NCHS and the Department of Health and Human Services on the overall directions and scope and content of the National Health Care Data System, in the context of the agenda set forth by the panel in its proposed strategy for implementation.

Recommendation 5-2: The panel recommends that an external technical committee of relevant experts be established during the planning and implementation phase to help plan and review the research needed to complete the proposed design; to identify the priorities for feasibility and research projects; and to monitor the progress made by NCHS in completing the research agenda and implementing the recommended design for a National Health Care Data System on schedule.

Recommendation 5-3: The panel recommends that the Department of Health and Human Services establish an ad hoc external high-level committee, comprised of persons who have distinguished themselves in the field of health care statistics, survey and sampling methods, and the provision of health services, to undertake a comprehensive review of the health care statistics activities throughout the department and report its findings directly to the secretary.

Recommendation 5-4: The panel recommends that the Department of Health and Human Services ensure that sufficient resources for maintaining capability for analysis and dissemination of the data collected be included in the resources allocated for the National Health Care Data System.

Recommendation 5-5: The panel recommends that adequate funds for operating the National Health Care Data System, estimated to be no less than $25-30 million per year, be included in the appropriated budget of the National Center for Health Statistics.

1

Introduction

Health care in the United States has become an extremely complex and expensive activity. Over the past several years, several important changes have been taking place in its delivery and financing; more changes are expected in the future in a continuing effort to meet the health care needs of the population at affordable costs. Clearly we need, now more than ever before, relevant and timely data to guide policy makers in making informed decisions regarding the health status of our nation and the effectiveness and efficiency of its health care delivery system. Unfortunately, for a variety of reasons, existing sources are unable to address fully a number of areas of health policy interest and are capable of providing only part of the information needed to evaluate changes in the organization, financing, and delivery of health care. Current surveys are inadequate, for example, in their coverage of emerging sites of medical care; in measuring the impact of change on the quality, effectiveness, and outcome of medical care; in tracking persons across health care settings; and in addressing the health care needs of the poor, minorities, and those without adequate health insurance.

Data are needed to measure the degree of shift from traditional to alternative health care settings and to provide national estimates for types of care delivered in these new settings, in order to continue to provide basic information on the supply and use of health services and health care technology. Data obtained from existing surveys are becoming less definitive as patients and treatments shift to other settings.

There is need also to assess the impact of changes, such as the introduction of new technologies in the practice of medicine, and to assess the change in the health outcomes that are brought about by modifications in financing and organization of such care. Data are needed on the differences in health outcomes between different geographic locations of surgery or other care in terms of subsequent institutionalization, mortality, or illness; differences in outcome from alternative treatments or technologies employed for the same diagnosis; and the impact of declining inpatient lengths of stay, for various diagnoses, on subsequent readmission, other care, and health outcomes. To be responsive to those needs and to others in the future, the statistical design for our data systems must have the flexibility, which they do not now have, to adapt to changes in the health care system as they occur.

Recognizing that our national data systems have been unable to keep pace with the changes occurring in the health care system in the past decade, the National Center for Health Statistics (NCHS), in the U.S. Department of Health and Human Services (DHHS), has developed plans for revision, expansion, and coordination of their data collection activities on health care utilization that currently are carried out in separate, independently designed, national provider-based[1] surveys. They have named this group of data collection activities the National Health Care Survey.

PANEL'S CHARGE AND ITS APPROACH

To obtain guidance in the development of national health care data for the 1990s and the decades to come, the director of NCHS requested that the National Research Council through its Committee on National Statistics and the Board on Health Care Services of the Institute of Medicine convene a panel of experts to evaluate its plan for the National Health Care Survey. The Panel on the National Health Care Survey held its first meeting in February 1990.

In order to evaluate the proposed plan for a National Health Care Survey, the panel was asked to carry out two major tasks:

(1) Identify the principal current and future needs for health care data by public and private policy makers, health care providers, health service researchers, and others and

(2) Determine the extent to which the proposed survey can meet identified needs for data given the statistical aspects of the survey such as sample design, sample size, data collection methods, and data sets.

---

[1] Throughout this report, use of the term *provider* includes both the individual health care provider and the facility or service setting where health service is provided.

In formulating its recommendations, the panel found it necessary to consider more than just the four provider surveys currently included in the center's plans for the National Health Care Survey (the center's formal plan is reproduced in Appendix A). The panel's consideration therefore included the other data systems of the center, such as the National Health Interview Survey, within the umbrella of the integrated design framework, as well as issues of a more general and broad nature than those outlined above. The panel also considered it important to address some of the basic issues concerning the internal capacity of the NCHS, the need for increased collaboration and integration of data systems among the DHHS agencies, and the efficient and coordinated use of resources in the development and analysis of health care statistics within DHHS.

To address its charge in a systematic manner, the panel decided early in its deliberations to obtain the views of a wide group of users, policy makers, and other interested parties. As a first step in this direction, an informal survey of users was conducted. Focused group interviews were conducted of selected federal health officials, legislative staff, researchers, and state vital and health statisticians. The interviews followed a protocol developed to ensure that all issues were discussed during the interviews. Detailed notes of the interviews were prepared for the panel's review and discussion. Views of more than 70 people representing a wide variety of organizations were obtained in this manner. The findings of the survey of users and the interview guide used for the group meetings are summarized in Chapter 2 and appear in full in Appendix B. The panel also obtained the views of users through oral presentations at its meetings; representatives of the various federal agencies that have an interest in health care data and others were invited to express their needs for data and to comment on their use of the existing data systems.

The panel reviewed an extensive body of material: planning documents; internal memoranda; relevant internal documents related to design, redesign plans, and other material provided by NCHS and other department officials during the course of the study; as well as historical documents and publications relating to the surveys under consideration. Literature on the changes in the health care system in the United States also was reviewed.

In response to its charge, the panel developed a set of recommendations for the content, coverage, and design for a data system for this decade and into the next century. Some aspects of the panel's proposals are similar to those contained in the center's current plans, with some modifications and expansion. Other proposals, however, reflect important conceptual and operational recommendations that go beyond the current plans and are intended to enhance the capability of the data system to serve the nation's needs for statistical information about its health care system. Although the modifications to the plan that are proposed cannot be accomplished immediately, the panel believes that the center should begin the phased implementation of these recommendations without delay. The panel's proposals are intended to provide a comprehensive, integrated, yet realistic package that should be phased in as a whole.

ORGANIZATION OF THE REPORT

The report is organized in a manner responsive to the charge. Chapter 2 is a discussion of the changing health care delivery system in the United States and the implications for needs for comprehensive and current data to monitor the changes, evaluate their effectiveness and guide development of health policy.

Chapter 3 presents the panel's review and critique of the center's plan for an integrated National Health Care Survey in its present stage of development and the panel's recommendations for modifications and expansion in the areas of coverage and content of the survey, the benefits and limitations of the center's design, and identification of areas that need further investigation.

Chapter 4 lays out the panel's recommended approach toward an integrated National Health Care Data System and presents the panel's strategy for implementation by the year 2000. This chapter states the panel's conclusions about the current plan, presents recommendations about new directions, and suggests steps and a timetable by which such a survey design might be put in place.

Finally, Chapter 5 highlights some basic issues of capacity, coordination, and resource considerations about the health care activities of DHHS.

Although the principal intent of this report is to address the specific concerns of NCHS regarding the optimal approach for gathering needed data about the health care system, the panel is hopeful that the report will provide guidance to a wider audience responsible for federal health care policy, and in general contribute toward development of an efficient and cost-effective data base for monitoring the quality, access to, and costs of health care in the United States.

2

Data Needs for a Changing Health Care Delivery System

To establish what improvements and innovations in national data sources might best be pursued and with what priorities, policy makers must first appreciate the diverse features and trends in the health care arena today and the critical questions they pose. To identify current and future needs for health care data, they must grasp the changes that have led to the present configuration of the health care delivery system and the challenges it faces. These involve shifts and innovations in the organization of services, the relationships among different service settings, financing arrangements, and the coverage of the population—and, ultimately, changes in the health of that population.

This chapter briefly reviews key features of and developments in health care that provide the framework for considering reform of national health data sources—both the proposed National Health Care Survey and broader data systems as well. The bedrock issues relate to costs, access, and quality; cutting across them are trends relating to demographics and socioeconomic factors, health and disease, technology, human resources, and related social, legal, and ethical questions. Because space limitations prohibit a historical overview, the focus is on current factors and circumstances; readers interested in details of the evolution of the U.S. health care system are referred to Somers and Somers (1961), Torrens (1978), Starr (1982), and Aaron (1991b). A survey of users of national health care statistics undertaken by the panel is also described briefly; Appendix B has a more complete discussion. The last section returns to the subject of data sources and systems and their desirable characteristics.

THREE CRITICAL ISSUES IN HEALTH CARE

Health care pundits often characterize the goals of the U.S. health care system as being access for all to high- (or at least acceptable) quality care at affordable (or reasonable) cost. The nation's present system meets none of the goals of access, quality, and cost consistently, and certainly not simultaneously, and some observers regard health care in this country as in crisis because of the extent to which these goals are not being accomplished (Aaron, 1991a). Furthermore, it is perhaps a commonplace to note the immense complexity of U.S. society and its health care system; nonetheless, many social, economic, and technological factors heavily influence what can, and cannot, be done to achieve progress toward those three goals.

Health researchers and policy makers therefore have a compelling need for more and better data on a considerable number of issues if they are to make sense of current problems and the options available to address them. The issues and data presented below are intended to illustrate some of that complexity and thereby to underscore the difficulties facing those who must design and implement programs to make data available in a timely way.

Costs and Expenditures

A pressing issue confronting the health care system today is the continued upward escalation in health care expenditures and costs of care. The figures are compelling (Office of National Cost Estimates, 1990; Levit et al., 1991; Aaron, 1991b). A quarter-century ago, national health care expenditures just exceeded $40 billion, or about 6 percent of the gross national product (GNP). At the start of the 1990s, outlays stood at more than $600 billion, or 12 percent of GNP. To be precise, expenditures in 1991 were $670.9 billion (12.3 percent of GNP). Estimates for 1992, 1995, and 2000 have been put, respectively, at $809.0 billion (13.4 percent), $1,072.7 (14.7 percent) and $1,615.9 (16.4 percent) (Office of National Health Statistics, 1991).

These levels of expenditures well outstrip those of other industrialized countries. For example, in 1989 the per capita expenditure on health in the United States was $2,354, a figure that exceeded per capita spending for Canada by 40 percent, for Germany by 91 percent, for the United Kingdom by 182 percent, and for Turkey by 1,245 percent (Schieber et al., 1991). *Rates of real growth* in health care spending for Organisation for Economic Cooperation and Development (OECD) countries for the past three decades are not very different, however, suggesting that the United States has outspent the rest of the world for almost the last half-century (J. Newhouse, personal communication, 1991).

These disparities in spending have not translated into better (or sometimes even equivalent) coverage of the population or better health outcomes as reflected in standard indices (Schieber and Poullier, 1988, 1989; NCHS, 1990, 1991). For example, in terms of infant and perinatal mortality rates, the United States ranks twentieth and sixteenth, respectively, in a comparison among 24 OECD countries (Schieber et al., 1991). The picture is not much better for life expectancy, in which the United States ranks sixteenth and seventeenth for female and male life expectancy at birth, respectively. An interesting exception is life expectancy at 80 years of age, in which the United States ranks second after Canada and Iceland (female) and Canada, Japan, and Switzerland (male). One analysis of 10 Western industrialized nations, which compared them in terms of extent of primary health services, levels of 12 standard health indices, and people's satisfaction with their health care systems, found that ratings for the United States on these variables were generally low (as were those of West Germany) in contrast to Canada, Sweden, and the Netherlands, which had generally high ratings (Starfield, 1991).

Virtually every part of the health care sector has experienced increases in expenditures for care—both the private and the public sectors (especially Medicare); both fee-for-service and prepaid capitated systems; and both inpatient and outpatient care. For example, spending for hospital care increased 9.3 percent between 1987 and 1988 (to just under $212 billion); spending for physician services increased 13.1 percent (to just over $105 billion) (Office of National Cost Estimates, 1990). Furthermore, costs to third-party payers (i.e., insured costs) and to patients and families (i.e., out-of-pocket payments) have grown; for the latter, for instance, the increase between 1987 and 1988 was more than 10 percent (Office of National Cost Estimates, 1990).

Employer-based insurance is the primary way health care is financed in the United States. Increases in employers' group health premiums have been steep in recent years: 20 to 24 percent in 1989 alone by two different estimates (Cantor et al., 1991; Sullivan and Rice, 1991). An average premium increase of only 14 percent for 1990 (Sullivan and Rice, 1991) may, however, partly reflect emerging changes in the health insurance picture: a shift toward health plans with utilization management requirements, more health maintenance organizations (HMOs) and preferred provider organization (PPO) arrangements, and growth in point-of-service plans, as well as greater cost-sharing by employees (in the form of higher proportions of total monthly premiums or higher deductibles or copayment rates).

In short, the rise in what the nation spends on health—in percentage terms well in excess of the rate of inflation—seems so inexorable that it generates calls for rationing (Aaron and Schwartz, 1984, 1990; Callahan, 1987, 1990). Equally firm counterarguments are advanced, however, to the effect that improving the efficiency of the health care system and reducing the provision of unnecessary and inappropriate care would help to keep the rate of expenditure growth under control and thereby forestall the need for rationing (Brook and Lohr, 1986; Wennberg, 1990a). Widely differing connotations of the term rationing—as "social allocation," as "principled rationalization," and as "cost-effective retrenchment" (Brown, 1991, p. 30)—tend to inhibit clear communication and complicate the debate.

Many explanations for the upward spiral of expenditures have been advanced. Among them are: the effect of third-party insurance coverage in insulating people from the true costs of care; the ever-increasing sophistication of medical technologies; the changing demographics of the population; the ability of health care providers to generate demand for their services; lack of certain knowledge about the efficacy, effectiveness, and appropriateness of health care interventions; and rising expectations of patients and others about what health care can (or ought to be able to) do to extend life and enhance the quality of that life (or both). One of the challenges that must be met by data sources of the 1990s and beyond is to overcome the lacunae in information that keep researchers and decision makers from understanding better which, if any, of these explanations are the most plausible and amenable to change.

The nation has seen many attempts to control rising expenditures. The shift from cost-reimbursement strategies for Medicare reimbursement of hospital care to the diagnosis-related group (DRG) prospective payment system for Medicare is one of the more dramatic examples. Direct controls on charges (price controls, fee schedules for physicians) have also been or will be tried. Efforts to constrain the use of services, as a means of controlling costs, take several forms; higher levels of cost-sharing imposed by third-party payers and various approaches to utilization management and managed care are among the more prevalent. Incentives to use more ambulatory (rather than inpatient) care also share the goal of controlling costs.

Even the HMO movement can be seen in part as an effort to deal with the use and costs of care better than the traditional fee-for-service system has done (Luft, 1981, 1991). More broadly, some observers believe that managed care—itself an imprecisely defined and understood term variously embracing utilization management (IOM, 1989a), traditional and hybrid versions of HMOs and PPOs, and case management of high-risk patients—offers a mechanism for constraining use and expenditures.

The implications of these kinds of changes for data surveys and sources are many. They include the need for better systems for classifying and coding information on a large number of variables: sites and settings of care; personnel delivering care; types of care (with greater specificity than is available today for, as examples, procedures, drugs, diagnostic tests, and other technologies); charges for care; and costs of care.[1] To have better data of these sorts, and to be able to track them over time and aggregate them across sources, those responsible for data collection must come to agreement on several issues. These matters include, in particular: (1) the minimum number of data elements necessary to convey specific and aggregate cost and expenditures data adequately and to link them to relevant populations and providers and (2) the operational definitions of those data elements.

Access to Care

Access to care refers essentially to the ability of persons needing health services to recognize that need and to seek and obtain the appropriate care in a timely way. Appropriate care can be thought of as necessary and effective care that can reasonably be expected to make a difference in the health and well-being of those receiving it; in other words, it should maintain or improve the health status and quality of life of individuals and populations.

The services of interest must be broadly conceived:

- primary care, including health promotion and preventive and screening services;

- specialized secondary and tertiary services, including inpatient care of the full range of acute and chronic illness, outpatient and inpatient care for mental and emotional disorders and for alcohol and drug abuse problems; dental care; rehabilitation therapy; and the like;

- various forms of sociomedical services—home health care, adult day care, and related social services—that are aimed at maintaining ill or disabled individuals in their homes and communities and out of institutions;

- long-term institution-based care; and

- hospice and respite care and similar specialized services that may be provided at the end of life.

Tracking the need for and use of this broad array of services presents a major challenge for the nation's data systems. Detecting the *unmet* need for

---

[1] As to the latter two points, economists correctly distinguish charges and costs on both theoretical and empirical grounds; policy makers and researchers often ignore the distinctions at some peril to appropriate analysis and interpretation of data.

and lack of appropriate use of such services is an even more daunting task. Among the major difficulties are defining, classifying, and assessing the populations of interest in appropriate ways.

Poor access to care for at least some groups in U.S. society has been an ever-present problem. It was recognized in the mid-twentieth century as sufficiently acute for elderly and poor people (especially families with dependent children) that the Medicare and Medicaid programs were enacted.

In terms of providing insurance coverage to now more than 30 million elderly people, the Medicare program has been a remarkable success. Generally, the elderly enjoy better access to care, in the form of insurance coverage, than any other age group in the nation (IOM, 1990c; Aaron, 1991b; NCHS, 1991). Nevertheless, compared with employment-based private insurance, the Medicare program *alone* gives less protection against devastating out-of-pocket spending by older Americans because it does not cover prescription drugs and does not cap copayment costs for covered services (CBO, 1991b). Only Medicare enrollees with employment-based retiree health benefits (about 30 percent), with so-called medigap supplemental policies (31 percent), or Medicaid benefits (18 percent) are protected to some degree from the risk of catastrophic out-of-pocket costs.

By contrast, individuals and families with low incomes are not well covered by the federal-state Medicaid program. The Pepper Commission (the U.S. Bipartisan Commission on Comprehensive Health Care, 1990), for example, cites figures indicating that only 42 percent of people in poverty—and only about 75 percent of those in extreme poverty (those with family incomes below 25 percent of the poverty line)—were covered by Medicaid in 1987. Various categorical exclusions and remarkable variations in eligibility rules across the states have kept a wide range of people out of the program, even if they are penniless. Some of these features are changing, however, as Congress has attempted to expand eligibility at least for pregnant women and young children and for those who experience an increase in income because of return to employment.

Complicating the picture of access to health care for the poor is that Medicaid itself devotes increasing fractions of its resources to reimburse elderly people for long-term nursing home care. Of all Medicaid outlays in 1988, for example, 37 percent were for nursing home care, and these accounted for more than 44 percent of all expenditures on such care that year (Office of National Cost Estimates, 1990). In 1990, as a fraction of the total spending on personal health care services in Medicaid, the outlays for nursing home care were just over 33 percent, or about 92 percent of the combined Medicare-Medicaid spending for this type of service (Office of National Health Statistics, 1991).

Still, today's most visible access problem lies with the 35 million or so people who lack any (or at least adequate) health insurance: 40 million in

1996 by one estimate (Aaron, 1991a).[2] This group tends to be disproportionately poor. Of the approximately 32 million uninsured in 1987, for example, 30 percent came from families with incomes between 0 and 100 percent of the federal poverty level (and 32 percent from families between 101 and 200 percent), compared with 21 percent from families with incomes greater than 300 percent of poverty (U.S. Bipartisan Commission on Comprehensive Health Care, 1990). As a percentage of all people in various income groups, 32 percent of those with annual family incomes between 0 and 100 percent of poverty were uninsured, compared with 6 percent of those with incomes greater than 300 percent of poverty (U.S. Bipartisan Commission on Comprehensive Health Care, 1990). In short, about 15 percent of the population faces severe constraints on their ability to receive appropriate and timely care of the sorts outlined above. Although eventually they may be able to acquire services for acute or chronic illnesses, those services may be sporadic, fragmented across providers, unnecessarily delayed, and of questionable quality.

The issue is especially serious for children, particularly those in uninsured families not sufficiently poor to be eligible for Medicaid. That is, the uninsured are disproportionately young; more than a quarter are children under 18. More concretely, about 83 percent of all children through age 17 were covered by some health insurance plan or Medicaid in 1988, but only 72 percent of children in families with annual incomes under $10,000 were so covered, compared with 92 percent of children in families with incomes over $40,000 (Bloom, 1990).

Lack of or inadequate insurance coverage—and attendant high or insurmountable out-of-pocket costs—are not the only hindrances to access to and appropriate use of care. Various other problems associated with residence (e.g., rural areas, inner cities) can be cited (although they differ by site). For example, some residents of rural areas not adjacent to metropolitan areas may face long-distance travel to sites of care, small or inadequately staffed and equipped facilities, and a dearth of physicians (especially specialists).[3] People in the inner cities may have to cope with overcrowded

---

[2]Estimates of the number of uninsured people in this nation vary considerably, depending partly on definitions and partly on time frames. The Pepper Commission cites about 31.5 million (15 percent of the nonelderly) who had no health insurance in 1987; Ries (1991) cites about 33.9 million (14 percent) in 1989. Short (1990) puts the number of people lacking coverage for all or part of 1987 at 48 million (about 20 percent of the population); more timebound estimates suggest that 36 million people were completely uninsured in the first quarter of 1987, 34 million in last quarter.

[3]The issue of whether rural areas are underserved by physicians, or by physicians in specialty practice compared with primary practice, is a tangled one. It is discussed in more detail in the section on human resources below.

facilities and clinics, fraudulent "Medicaid mills," and the lack of physicians able to communicate in languages other than English.

In addition to these problems, access to care may be further limited for specific population groups. These include ethnic and racial minorities, non-English-speakers, people with various impairments and disabilities (physical handicaps, blindness, deafness), people with various stigmatizing conditions, such as the acquired immune deficiency syndrome (AIDS), and homeless people.

Finally, certain other features of the current health care landscape impinge on people's access to care. Very critical may be the current medical malpractice and liability climate, in which fear of being sued or the need to pay high malpractice premiums, or both, drives physicians out of certain high-risk specialties. This is especially true for obstetrics or at least the delivery of obstetric care (IOM, 1989b).

Low rates of reimbursement for physicians' services are also declared to be a barrier to access. This is a significant issue at least for Medicaid, where low fees are one tactic for (presumably) controlling expenditures, insofar as physicians will refuse to take any (or at least new) Medicaid patients. Some observers are also concerned that physician payment reform in Medicare (national fee schedules, control on volume of services through volume performance standards, and limits on balance billing) will, first, drive some payments for services below those typical even for Medicaid and, second, negatively affect access for the elderly to key health services (AARP, 1991b).

Quality of Care

A recent Institute of Medicine report has defined quality of care as "the degree to which *health services* for *individuals and populations* increase the likelihood of desired *health outcomes* and are consistent with current professional knowledge" (IOM, 1990c: 21, emphasis added). The report characterized problems with quality of care as stemming from three sources: overuse of unnecessary and inappropriate care; underuse of needed and effective care; and poor technical and interpersonal performance on the part of health care providers. The emphasis on health services, individuals and populations, and outcomes—plus the breadth of questions that flow from overuse, underuse, and poor care—highlight the extraordinary set of topics that standard surveys must consider in measuring and monitoring quality of care.

Attention to quality of care and to the evaluation and improvement of health care has waxed and waned over the years, often in response to programs intended to deal with expenditures on and access to care. There has been some resurgence in interest in quality of care, quality assurance, and continuous quality improvement in recent years (*Health Affairs*, 1988; *Inquiry*, 1988; Lohr et al., 1988; Goldfield and Nash, 1989; Palmer et al., 1991). Strenuous efforts to stem the use of health care services and control expenditures prompt various interest groups (e.g., health care providers, patients) to predict harmful consequences for the quality of health care. A case in point is the predictions of harm to quality of care for Medicare beneficiaries secondary to the implementation of a DRG-based prospective payment system—predictions not borne out to date (Kahn et al., 1990a, 1990b). Nevertheless, many participants in health care delivery, as well as many patients, express concern about the quality of the care they deliver or receive now or will in the future.

Quality of care is often seen as having three dimensions: (1) the so-called structural characteristics of providers and practitioners (various organizational and professional factors); (2) the process of care (or what is done to and for patients with respect to diagnosis, treatment, rehabilitation, and palliation); and (3) the outcomes of care. These three dimensions are important in traditional approaches to quality assessment and assurance (Donabedian, 1966, 1980, 1982, 1985) as well as in newer approaches involving continuous quality improvement and total quality management (Batalden and Buchanan, 1989; Berwick, 1989; Berwick et al., 1990). The last-named dimension—variously termed outcomes, health status, health-related quality of life, patient well-being, and the like—has gained considerable attention and utility in recent years (Brook et al., 1976; Gilford, 1988; Ellwood, 1988; Lohr, 1988; Tarlov et al., 1989).

Most experts in this area agree that understanding the relationship between the process of care and outcomes of that care is essential, and they lament the striking lack of information that might demonstrate those linkages. Generally, the process of care—that is, the services rendered—has been and is easier to define, document, and evaluate than are outcomes of care. As a consequence, existing data systems do not include adequate indicators of outcomes that could be used to evaluate quality.

What is needed to measure this dimension of quality of care—i.e., the outcomes of care, or the individual's health status—adequately? Health status is a complex, multidimensional construct reflecting significant aspects of an individual's or a population's life circumstances. It usually incorporates five major areas of interest—physical health, mental health, social functioning, role functioning, and general health perceptions. Some experts add pain as a key domain; some add cognitive functioning, or energy and vitality, or both. The literature may differ somewhat in the typology of these (or related) domains, but the basic classifications are becoming relatively standard (Katz, 1987; Ware, 1987; Lohr and Ware, 1987; Patrick and Erickson, 1988; Lohr, 1989; Mosteller and Falotico-Taylor, 1989; Patrick and Bergner, 1990).

A partial list of variables pertinent to domains of health-related quality of life (which some regard as synonymous with health status and others take to be broader) includes: survival and life expectancy; various symptoms, such as pain; numerous physiologic states, such as blood pressure or serum glucose levels; physical function states of many sorts, for instance, mobility and ambulation, sensory functioning (such as seeing or hearing), sexual functioning, a range of capacities relating to impairment, disability, and handicap, and specific measures of activities of daily living; emotional and cognitive function status, such as anxiety and depression or positive well-being; perceptions about present and future health; and satisfaction with health care.

Aspects of quality of care other than outcomes must also be considered. One is the continuity of care, which implies that one must evaluate the flow of illness and wellness, and the services sought and rendered, through an entire episode of care (rather than in a single encounter) and thus across time and settings of care. A second, related factor is coordination of care. Yet another is the satisfaction of both the recipient and the provider with the care rendered, a facet of health care that some place directly in any listing of outcomes; satisfaction can in turn relate to a broad set of questions concerning accessibility, availability, and costs of care in addition to ratings of the technical and interpersonal performance of clinicians and institutions. Adequately addressing this inventory of information in data systems of the future poses an immense challenge to policy makers and researchers alike.

HEALTH CARE REFORM

The calls for health care reform and the proposals emanating from several blue-ribbon panels in recent years have centered on finding ways to solve particular problems of access to care (especially those of the uninsured and underinsured). The aim is to overcome the access barriers without exacerbating the problems of costs or undermining the quality of care received.

A peculiarity of the problem of being uninsured in the United States is that most people in this situation are in families with at least one employed worker—a seeming anomaly, insofar as the great bulk of health insurance in this country is employer-based. Perhaps not surprisingly, therefore, the main ideas being advanced generally call for the enactment of various kinds of mandates for employers to offer at least basic insurance plans to their employees or to contribute to a public-sector pool that will cover such individuals (ideas generally referred to as "play or pay"). Among the better known proposals, for instance, are those emanating from the Pepper Commission. These would, among other things, require all individuals to obtain health care coverage from their employers or from a public program, the latter a new version of Medicaid to cover the unemployed and the poor (U.S. Bipartisan Commission on Comprehensive Health Care, 1990).

These kinds of proposals—including ones being advanced by the American Federation of Labor and Congress of Industrial Organizations, by the American Medical Association, by various health policy and health economics experts, by business coalitions, and politicians—are relatively middle-of-the-road, politically speaking. As noted, they would either require compulsory private insurance through employers or direct that employers either provide private insurance to employees or pay an equivalent tax, with government insuring nonworkers and the poor (Blendon and Edwards, 1991; Haglund, 1991; *JAMA*, 1991). More radical or reform-minded proposals appear to favor, on one hand, a Canadian-style national health program (Marmor and Mashaw, 1990; Woolhandler and Himmelstein, 1989, 1991; Himmelstein and Woolhandler, 1989) and, on the other hand, competition-oriented approaches or programs to require individuals to acquire their own health insurance and receive tax credits for doing so (Butler, 1991).

Debates over the attempt to ration Medicaid care in Oregon (the Oregon Basic Health Services Act) (Fox and Leichter, 1991; Grannemann, 1991; Sipes-Metzler, 1991) underscore the immense diversity of proposals now being aimed at health care reform and the appreciable emotional overlay that accompanies them (Brown, 1991; Callahan, 1991; Etzioni, 1991). Widening interest in what can be learned for the United States from other countries may help to break what some perceive to be a health care policy gridlock (*Health Affairs*, 1991; Peet, 1991; Reinhardt, 1991; Starfield, 1991).

The directions that health care reform is likely to take, as reflected in these kinds of ideas, are not at all clear. The implications for data survey and collection efforts are also murky. Those designing and implementing such survey programs will surely need to give strict attention to (1) key elements of health care financing and reimbursement proposals or legislated strategies for reform; (2) measures of expenditures, access, outcomes, and quality of care; (3) providers of health care, broadly defined; and (4) the populations affected by such strategies, particularly children, ethnic minorities, and the elderly (and the very old). Cutting across these points is the requirement that planning and implementation of reform require respectable, comprehensive data that still permit a focus on special groups.

OTHER FACTORS INFLUENCING HEALTH CARE POLICY AND DATA NEEDS

Demographics and Socioeconomic Factors

The evolving nature of U.S. society poses notable challenges to health care delivery. Most significant, perhaps, is what is called the "graying of

America": the population is becoming older, on average, and the elderly population itself is aging. Data from the mid-1980s suggests, for instance, an increase in the population age 65 and older of 75 percent between 1960 and 1986, compared with a 30-percent increase among those under age 65 (NCHS, 1989). Between 1987 and 2030, those under age 20 are projected to drop as a percentage of the total population from 29 to 24 percent and those age 20 to 64 to drop from 59 to 56 percent; by contrast, those age 65 and older will increase from 12 to 21 percent (Waldo et al., 1989). The oldest elderly (those age 85 and older)—typically the sickest—constitute the fastest-growing portion of the elderly population (Gilford, 1988).

Other factors and trends are significant as well. With respect to the elderly, the numerical predominance of women over men is striking. Furthermore, the vast majority of the elderly (and hence elderly women) live in the community, and of those about one-third live alone. Of those residing in nursing homes, most are very old (age 85 and older) and female. Poverty rates among the elderly have been declining in recent years, but even so about one in three elderly people was below 150 percent of the poverty line in the mid-1980s (Special Committee on Aging, 1987-1988).

The proportion of the total population accounted for by immigrants and nonimmigrant minorities is growing. Toward the end of the 1980s, the racial composition of the U.S. population was about 84 percent white, 12 percent black, 8 percent Hispanic (of any race), 3 percent Asian and Pacific Islander, and 1 percent American Indian and Alaskan native (NCHS, 1991). The Hispanic and Asian populations have both grown considerably since 1980 (in both absolute and percentage terms), the former about equally from immigration and natural increase and the latter almost entirely from immigration (NCHS, 1991).

The contrasts between minority populations, particularly blacks and Hispanic groups, and the majority (white) population with respect to socioeconomic and health factors are dramatic (U.S. DHHS, 1991a). Virtually every health status and health utilization measure shows those subgroups as disadvantaged relative to whites; in some cases (e.g., life expectancy and infant mortality for blacks), the disparities are widening. The problems are so acute that the DHHS secretary has made minority health issues a top priority for the 1990s.

Apart from factors relating to age and ethnicity, the health care sector may be affected by trends in family income and makeup. One consideration is the growth in the number of families in poverty. The rise in the number of children in poverty is especially stark (Johnson et al., 1991): between 1979 and 1989, child poverty rates increased by 21 percent; one in five children currently lives in poverty; children have almost twice the likelihood of being poor as any other age group; and the younger the child, the greater the chance of being poor.

Likewise, both the lack of formation of and the breakup of stable families—through divorce, separation, and out-of-wedlock births, for instance—contribute to the growth of single-parent families and families in which the single parent may herself be barely out of childhood. Homeless people, an extremely heterogeneous group that can range from functioning families temporarily down on their luck to mentally ill individuals who have been discharged from institutions to the community, is another population for which the current health care system has little to offer (IOM, 1988; Brickner et al., 1990). Various types of nontraditional households, such as homosexual couples for whom obtaining conventional health insurance may be a problem, are yet another element of society that poses challenges to health care delivery and policy. (The predicament is exacerbated by the loss of private health insurance among homosexual men with AIDS, although this may be more a consequence of loss of employment owing to sickness than to exclusionary insurance practices per se—Kass et al., 1991). Nevertheless, the difficulties posed to survey and surveillance systems of the 1990s and beyond by these extremely differing views of "families"[4] are profound.

Health and Disease

The causes of death, illness, and disability in this country, as in all industrialized countries and many industrializing nations, have changed significantly in the twentieth century. In broad terms across the U.S. population, a number of infectious diseases have come under control in the past 50 years or can now be cured. Because these were often diseases of the young, life expectancy has risen.

Chronic illnesses have taken the place of infectious disease as the leading causes of death and disability. They are increasingly prevalent because of the aging of the population and increasingly complex as greater numbers of people develop multiple chronic problems. Furthermore, the numbers of people suffering various disabilities—owing to genetic disorders, chronic

---

[4]A recent compilation of definitions of *family*, for documenting how nontraditional families may be recognized for purposes of bereavement and sick leave, extension of health benefits, and similar matters underscores the variability in how this term is understood and used (legally, socially, and emotionally). One definition from California is "a unit of intimate transacting and interdependent persons who share the same values and goals, responsibility for decisions and resources, and a commitment to one another over time"; another has it that a family is "a unit of interdependent and interacting persons, related together over time by strong social and emotional bonds and/or by ties of marriage, birth, and adoption, whose central purpose is to create, maintain, and promote the social, mental, physical and emotional development and well-being of each of its members." Similarly, a definition from New York holds that "a more realistic . . . view [is that] a family includes two adult lifetime partners whose relationship is long-term and characterized by an emotional and financial commitment and interdependence" (all cited in National Gay and Lesbian Task Force Policy Institute, 1990-1991).

illnesses and the aging process, improved treatment of previously life-threatening wounds and injuries suffered in wartime, and various types of other injuries such as automobile accidents—are also growing. The conditions themselves are more complex than the infectious diseases they have replaced, and people live longer with them, often with a poor quality of life (IOM, 1991d). These and related developments all pose likely increasing demands for home health, rehabilitative, and related types of care—and for better data on incidence, prevalence, measures of severity and comorbidity, impairment and disability, and quality of life (Stoto, 1992).

Superimposed on this basic pattern of the incidence and prevalence of acute and chronic conditions is a set of sociomedical conditions that have had or threaten to have great impact on the need for health care. The AIDS epidemic has perhaps been perceived as the most menacing problem in recent years, for several reasons—its essentially 100-percent fatality rate, the rapid growth in the numbers and diversity of infected persons, the real and perceived threat to the nation's blood supply, and the biological diversity of the human immunosuppressive virus (HIV) itself.

Other significant health problems stem from the of use and abuse of illegal drugs, alcohol, and tobacco (U.S. DHHS, 1991a). Among these are (1) the use of crack cocaine and sequelae such as crack-addicted and developmentally affected babies and children of school age and (2) disability and premature death from automobile accidents involving alcohol abuse. The contribution of smoking to disease and premature death is well established; rates of smoking among certain populations (teenagers, women, and minorities) have not come down even in the face of that evidence. Interpersonal violence in the form of homicide and child and spouse abuse arise partly from some of the causes noted above and partly from the generally increasing levels of stress in U.S. society secondary to racial, economic, and other tensions. Finally, intrapersonal violence, that is, suicide and attempted suicide, is also on the rise, at least among teenagers and the elderly (Rosenberg et al., 1987; Meehan et al., 1991).

Healthy People 2000, the 1990 report of the secretary of DHHS outlining national health promotion and disease prevention objectives, is a partial response to these changing mortality and morbidity patterns and trends (U.S. DHHS, 1991a). It proffers three national health goals: increase the span of healthy life, lower health disparities among Americans, and provide access to preventive services for all Americans. These translate into perhaps 400 different objectives, and thus statistical series that will need to be monitored (Stoto, 1992)—an imposing task indeed.

Changing Values and Expectations

People's attitudes toward health and health care services have altered considerably in past years. Patients now expect to have a greater say in the decisions about how they shall be cared for. That is, they expect to be informed about all (reasonable) options open to them and about the expected benefits and risks of those options, so that they may express and exercise their own preferences for or against certain health states or the sequelae of different health care services.

These choices may be about care for essentially symptomatic (but not life-threatening) problems, such as the alternatives of surgery and "watchful waiting" for benign prostatic hypertrophy (Wennberg et al., 1987; Barry et al., 1988; Fowler et al., 1988). They may be about care for possibly life-threatening diseases, such as the alternatives of lumpectomy (with or without chemotherapy, hormonal therapy, or radiotherapy) or mastectomy for breast cancer (IOM, 1990a). Or they may be about care at the end of life, when the decision may be not to start, or not to continue, various extraordinary technologies that might prolong life at the significant expense of the quality of that life.

Regardless of the situation, however, patients more and more can be expected to want to exercise some autonomy about what is, or is not, done for them. For policy makers to be able to make sense of utilization (and hence expenditures) data as well as outcomes and quality-of-care data, those responsible for amassing that information will need to be increasingly sensitive to these issues. They will also need to design their data collection strategies to take patient preferences and autonomous actions stemming from those preferences adequately into account.

Technology, Innovation, and Biomedical Advance

One public policy goal immediately following World War II was to increase investment in biomedical research. Rapid increases in funding expanded substantially the scope and size of the National Institutes of Health and related funding of biomedical and clinical investigators. This funding and the simultaneous federal investment in the education of scientists resulted in tremendous advances in fundamental biology (molecular biology, neurobiology, genetics) and in the application of basic science to the prevention, diagnosis, and treatment of disease. Although some have criticized the emphasis on the development of halfway technologies such as dialysis and transplantation (Thomas, 1972), there is little doubt that these technologies have radically changed medical care (Altman and Blendon, 1979; Banta et al., 1981; Gelijns, 1991), as well as dramatically influenced the health and biomedical policy scene (IOM, 1991c). Moreover, issues concerning the conduct of and support for research and development of new technologies (the early innovation stages, for example) are being more carefully studied and debated (IOM, 1990-1992); more broadly, the field of technology assessment has received much attention in the last decade or two (OTA, 1982; IOM, 1985).

Developments during the past four decades cover virtually every segment of health care—that is, prevention, diagnosis, and treatment—and virtually every aspect of health and illness. Among the more dramatic achievements have been those related to life-threatening or fatal illness:[5] open heart surgery and bypass grafting; cardiac assist devices, including total artificial hearts; heart, lung, kidney, and liver transplants; and a vast array of pharmaceutical agents for medical and mental illnesses. Less visible but perhaps no less dramatic have been diagnostic steps: automated laboratories; computer-aided tomography (CAT) scans, magnetic resonance imaging (MRI), and positron emission tomography. In the prevention area, vaccines against a number of diseases (for example, hepatitis B and poliomyelitis) are bringing these diseases under greater control. Many impressive technologies come together in units such as those devoted to coronary care and neonatal intensive care. Finally, major breakthroughs can be expected in molecular biology, genetics, and bioengineering—the prospects of mapping and sequencing the human genome, for example, are monumental and daunting (CLS/NRC, 1991).

Initially, because of the cost, the reimbursement system, and the intensity of treatment, the hospital was the focus of placement for most of the new technology, and many of the nation's hospitals sought to acquire in as timely as way as possible the relevant equipment and professional staffs. This pattern is now changing in two ways. First, in the last two decades, automation, advances in anesthesia and surgical techniques and other technologies, and reimbursement and cost containment policies have stimulated the movement of certain types of technology out of the hospital setting. New facilities have emerged and grown to address this health care market. Second, assuming the evidence continues to lend credence to information that certain technologies (especially complex surgical procedures) require high volume and specific skills to reach acceptable levels of mortality, morbidity, and quality of care (Luft et al., 1987; OTA, 1988), greater regionalization of these technologies (typically in hospital settings) may well occur. Reshaping the hospital industry and developing vertical systems of care will also accelerate regionalization.

Many observers expect that the availability, coupled with the costs, of these existing and anticipated technologies will outstrip society's ability to provide their benefits to everyone. As noted in the discussions above concerning costs and access, demands are increasing to develop more rational approaches to distributing the benefits of technology. Apart from the many proposals for health care reform that have emerged in 1990-1991, other key steps include the expansion of outcomes and effectiveness research (Brook

---

[5]Two recent IOM studies have explored many issues relating to two expensive, life-saving technologies. One concerns end-stage renal disease (IOM, 1991a; Levinsky and Rettig, 1991), the other the total artificial heart (IOM, 1991b).

and Lohr, 1985; Ellwood, 1988; NCHSR, 1988; Roper et al., 1988; IOM, 1990d; Wennberg, 1990b). Development of clinical practice guidelines, for instance by the Agency for Health Care Policy and Research in the U.S. Public Health Service, by medical specialty societies, and by other groups is another indicator of public, payer, professional, and policy maker response to concerns about overuse or misuse of services, spiraling health care spending, and quality of care (Chassin, 1988; Brook, 1989, 1990, 1991; USPSTF, 1989; AMA, 1990a, 1990b; Audet et al., 1990; Fletcher and Fletcher, 1990; IMCARE, 1990; IOM, 1990b, 1992; Leape, 1990; Eddy, 1991, forthcoming; GAO, 1991).

Interest has grown in the last two decades regarding the distribution, cost, and use of the accelerating number of new as well as established technologies. Some data exist on these matters. For example, the American Hospital Association surveys in-hospital availability of certain devices such as CAT scans, MRIs, and lithotripsy; manufacturers have proprietary information on sales of drugs and devices; and information on procedures can be found in insurance claims systems. Furthermore, special studies and surveys (like those now conducted by and being planned for NCHS) can provide at least some cross-sectional information.

The fact remains, however, that there is a paucity of information on the quantity and distribution of specific technologies according to settings, types of practitioners, and similar variables, as well as on their use according to demographic and health characteristics of patients; no comprehensive national data are collected on technology use. For example, as many types of technologies shift from the hospital sector to the outpatient sector, information from insurance claims is less and less helpful in tracking their use, because of the less comprehensive and less reliable coding of information on ambulatory care claims—with the possible exception of coding for visits and procedures, when it is done with CPT-4 (Current Procedural Terminology) codes rather than ICD-9-CM (International Classification of Diseases, ninth version, clinical modification) codes. As another illustration, although the Medicare Part A and Part B files collectively provide the best single source of information on use of health care (in this case, of course, just for the elderly), they provide no information on outpatient use of prescribed medications—a source of considerable concern about quality of care and out-of-pocket spending for the elderly (for example, 16 percent of annual out-of-pocket spending between $1,000 and $2,000 is for prescription drugs—(AARP, 1991a).

Data that link diagnoses with use of technology are not generally available except from selected clinical data banks. Commonality of procedures coding is essential to permit full utilization of different data banks on the use of technology. Outcome and quality assessment require data on diagnosis, use of drugs, devices, and procedures.

Human Resources

Certain trends in the emergence and use of different types of health professionals have significant implications for data sources. Among the more traditional health professions—for example, medicine and nursing—a move away from general practice is clear, although if the distinction is made between primary care and specialty practice, the trend is not so distinct. For example, in 1970, about 15 percent of all physicians were in general and family practice (27 percent of those in office-based practice); in 1987, the figure was 9 percent (16 percent for office-based practice) (NCHS, 1991). However, categorizing all nonfederal allopathic physicians as primary care or specialty care physicians, with the former being all general and family practice, internal medicine, obstetrics/gynecology, and pediatrics, changes the picture somewhat. In 1975-1976, 45 percent of this group was in primary care, 50 percent in specialty care; in 1987-1988, the figures were 44 percent and 51 percent (Frenzen, 1991)—hardly a meaningful shift over time.

One lingering debate is the extent to which physicians (both primary care and specialists) have diffused into nonmetropolitan or rural areas. Evidence amassed by researchers at the RAND Corporation in the early 1980s suggested, for instance, that most rural residents were within a half-hour drive of most types of specialists (Williams et al., 1983) and that even in physician-poor states, half the towns of 30,000 to 50,000 residents had neurosurgeons (Newhouse et al., 1982; J. Newhouse, personal communication, 1991). The expectation was that the diffusion of specialists into rural areas would increase as the total physician supply grew. Other investigators (cited in Frenzen, 1991) have presented different data and arrived at different conclusions or predictions—chiefly that few physicians would (or did) move into the most rural areas of the country. Examining physician manpower data for 1976 to 1987 for 10 categories of urban-rural locations, Frenzen (1991) concludes that the supply of physicians increased everywhere in the country, but that the increase was more rapid in metropolitan counties and nonmetropolitan urbanized areas not adjacent to metropolitan statistical areas, leading to a widening over time between urban and rural areas in the availability of physicians. (The exception to this comment concerns osteopaths, who were relatively more likely to settle in rural areas than allopathic physicians, especially in those states traditionally hospitable to that profession).

Superimposed on these patterns is the growth in the numbers of, or demand for the services of, various types of health professionals, such as dentists, psychologists, speech therapists, physical therapists, nurse practitioners, nurse midwives, and physician assistants. Within this picture, however, is a marked shortage (perceived or real) of certain kinds of personnel, particularly nurses and technicians (IOM, 1989c; NCHS, 1991). Aiken and Mullinex (1987) and the Commission on Nursing (of the secretary of the DHHS) conclude that cyclical imbalances between the supply of and demand for nurses result from excess demand, not an insufficient supply of nurses (L. Aiken, personal communication, 1991). Notwithstanding this evidence, many people in the health care sector, as well as much of the public, believe that a nursing shortage exists (Harris-Wehling, 1990; Walker, 1990).

The emergence of new types of providers—nurse practitioners, nurse midwives, and physician assistants, for example—is another notable trend. These types of practitioners present a cost-effective alternative to physicians, with no discernable decrement in quality of care (OTA, 1986). As public policy shifts to permit the public to choose such providers, and as reimbursement to such health professionals from third-party payers expands, demand for and use of their services may well grow as well.

USERS OF HEALTH CARE DATA

The panel determined early in its deliberations that it needed to learn more about (1) the kinds of health care data that actual users of the National Center for Health Statistics provider surveys desired now or might want in the future, (2) their satisfaction (or lack of it) with the information currently in those surveys, and (3) their views on the reliability, validity, costs, and accessibility of those surveys. To that end, the panel acquired information from users through presentations at panel meetings and focus group interviews. The methods and findings of those data-gathering efforts are given in greater detail in Appendix B. This section briefly summarizes the results.

Data needs most frequently identified concerned, not surprisingly, the major health policy issues discussed earlier. Among the specific issues related to costs were expenditures for prescription drugs and long-term care. With respect to access, users were concerned about populations lacking insurance, the elderly (especially as regards long-term and home health care), children and adolescents, people in rural areas, and people with HIV infections. Other issues concerned the impact of changes in financing and reimbursement generally, the effects of the shift from inpatient hospital care to ambulatory settings, and the effects of prevention programs on health habits, lifestyles, and outcomes.

The users interviewed raised other points as well. One topic concerned the need for person-based data, not just provider-based data, so that analyses can be done on episodes of care and across multiple providers and settings. A second involved the large number of different types of providers that NCHS does not now survey. Third, some respondents criticized the high level of geographic aggregation of current survey data, indicating a desire for data for (or the ability to extrapolate to) smaller geographic regions (e.g., states, rural areas, and perhaps even counties or communities). A fourth issue involved specific subpopulations (minorities defined by ethnicity and race as well as groups classified according to age, health status, socioeconomic level, and similar variables). A final matter of great concern to the respondents interviewed was the desire to be able to link the various NCHS data bases with each other as well as with Health Care Financing Administration (HCFA) data, social security records, and other databases.

IMPLICATIONS FOR DATA SOURCES AND SYSTEMS

NCHS surveys have been, for decades, models of how to conduct complex national surveys in the health care field. Vast numbers of epidemiologic, health policy, and even effectiveness studies have relied, and must continue to rely, on information from the *Vital and Health Statistics* series and other NCHS publications. In recent years, agency staff have pioneered methods of applying composite health status measures to information such as from the National Health Interview Survey (Erickson et al., 1989). Yet the political and economic constraints under which the agency was forced to operate in the 1980s, which perhaps have led to many of the difficulties cited below and in other chapters, should not be underestimated.

Despite this admirable record, existing data sources that might be expected to provide at least some of the information needed to monitor and evaluate changes in the availability, financing, and quality of health care are rapidly becoming outdated and less comprehensive than is desirable. Often they do not cover the universe of providers and sites of health care; neither do they cover the universe of patients or potential users of health care. They lack sufficient information on exactly what services are provided and what the outcomes of those services are; they are inexact with respect to financial data (charges, costs, and expenditures); they are not timely; and at times they are inaccurate, incomplete, and unreliable. In short, current national data systems, when taken together, do not provide the information needed to allow researchers and policy makers to assess the effect of changes in financing, organization, and delivery of health care, or the impact of other social and economic trends, on the appropriateness, quality, costs, and outcomes of care.

Among the directions in which database systems will need to move are the following:

- Better insurance claims data from the fee-for-service system and analogs from the prepaid, capitated systems (and from hybrid systems), especially among people younger than age 65;

- More information on clinical services and physiologic outcomes from medical records;

- More information from patients (and their surrogates or proxies) on health-related quality of life, perceptions of health status, and satisfaction with care;

- Better information on how much is spent for treating particular types of patients with particular types of illnesses (both direct and indirect costs, including out-of-pocket costs); and

- More specific information on the services and technologies being given and used, and on the types of personnel providing them.

A recent IOM meeting convened to begin planning activities in the area of database development for clinical evaluation also brought to the fore several significant "logjam" issues (Lohr and Durch, 1991).[6] These are relevant for the planning of future NCHS surveys in general. Among the more salient were various technical aspects of data collection, data analyses, and data exchange; a myriad of legal issues (privacy and confidentiality, malpractice); use of data (e.g., clinical applications, feedback in quality-assurance programs, administrative and managerial applications); and the impact of reimbursement and financing on data collection and database development.

No single survey, information source, or data collection mechanism system is likely ever to meet all these criteria, address all these technical problems, or meet all users' needs. Collectively, however, they should be flexible enough to adapt to health care system changes as they occur and to meet special needs on an ad hoc basis. They must be able to record shifts in the health care delivery system and related industries, to register changes in policies at the national level and perhaps subnational level, and to document the impact of these shifts and policy changes on providers and patients alike. More technically speaking, they also need to be flexible enough to

---

[6]Participants seemingly agreed that *database* is a singularly elastic term. It was (and is) used to refer to such dissimilar sources of information as the following (examples in parentheses): computerized administrative files (Social Security and Internal Revenue Service files); insurance claims files in both the public sector (Medicare, Medicaid; Department of Veterans Affairs) and the private sector (the "big five" health insurance companies); provider records of all sorts (hospitals; managed care organizations and networks; pharmacies; laboratories); registries (for cancer [tumors], trauma, bone marrow transplant, end-stage renal disease); regulatory systems (state systems for reporting hospital adverse events and incidents; credentialing agencies; the National Practitioner Data Bank for malpractice reporting); secondary research databases (the Rand Corporation's Health Insurance Experiment); surveys (of the National Center for Health Statistics; of provider associations); and vital and health statistics (e.g., birth and death certificate files).

facilitate integration and linkage of data generated in special studies with those compiled in ongoing data systems.

The panel concludes that, for the NCHS surveys to be able to meet future demands for information related to all the health policy and environmental issues summarized in this chapter, they must be developed in a coordinated manner. That is, the continued uncoordinated development of new, discrete data systems in NCHS and throughout the department with different definitions, documentation, coding protocols, and little ability to be linked for analysis would be a serious mistake. In the panel's judgment, the overriding focus of the integrated National Health Care Survey should be to provide statistics on a continuous basis that reflect the state of health care in the United States with respect to the key dimensions of costs, access, availability, quality, and effectiveness—both now and through time. These and similar issues, especially as they relate to the National Health Care Survey, are taken up in succeeding chapters of this report.

3

Review of the NCHS Plan for the National Health Care Survey

OVERVIEW

As discussed in Chapter 2, major changes in the organization, financing, and delivery of health care have outpaced the capabilities of existing national health care surveys to provide relevant and timely data to monitor the health care of the nation and evaluate the impact of the changes in the system. Although extensive national data activities exist, they are not ideally designed to yield the kinds of data needed for monitoring and evaluating the changes occurring in the nation's health care system or for health policy analysis and development. (Brief descriptions of some of the national health data systems maintained by the U.S. Department of Health and Human Services are presented in Appendix C).

In an effort to be responsive to various emerging national health care issues and to the associated data needs, the National Center for Health Statistics (NCHS) in 1986 undertook a review of its existing surveys of health care providers. As a result of this review, NCHS has developed a plan for restructuring its existing health care provider surveys into a new National Health Care Survey with the aim of providing a more complete and useful picture than now exists of the medical care provided in the United States. The center's plan for the survey is described in the document entitled, "The National Health Care Survey" (reproduced in Appendix A). This document was supplemented by additional material provided by

NCHS as it became available as well as presentations to the panel by NCHS officials.

According to the plan, the proposed National Health Care Survey will build on the four existing health care provider surveys, which will be merged, expanded over time, and linked geographically with the National Health Interview Survey (NHIS). The provider surveys are the National Hospital Discharge Survey, the National Ambulatory Medical Care Survey, the National Nursing Home Survey, and the National Master Facility Inventory. Table 1 is a profile of the current survey design for the NCHS health care provider surveys and the National Health Interview Survey. The primary objective of this new survey will be "to produce annual data on the use of health care and the outcomes of care for the major sectors of the health care delivery system. These data will describe the patient population, medical care provided, financing, and provider characteristics" (see Appendix A). The NCHS proposes to implement the National Health Care Survey over a period of years as resources permit. The phased implementation of the new survey design began in 1988.

The proposed survey has four main features:

(1) The survey will be conducted on an annual basis to eliminate gaps in data and fluctuations in resource requirements;

(2) The types of providers and settings sampled would be expanded to include an array of additional sites of health care, such as hospital emergency and outpatient departments, ambulatory surgery centers, home health agencies, and hospices;

(3) Sampling designs will be revised. An integrated three-stage cluster design will be used in which providers would be sampled from a subsample of the primary sampling units (PSU)[1] of the National Health Interview Survey; and

(4) A capability would be developed to conduct routine and specialized patient follow-up studies to examine issues related to the outcome and subsequent use of medical care.

By expanding the types of providers surveyed and by adding a follow-up component, NCHS hopes to enhance the kind and amount of information currently available about health care events.

---

[1] For the first stage of sample design for the National Health Interview Survey in which the civilian noninstitutionalized population residing in the United States is sampled, the United States is considered to be a universe composed of approximately 1,900 geographically defined primary sampling units. A primary sampling unit consists of a county, small group of contiguous counties, or a metropolitan statistical area. The PSUs collectively cover the 50 states and the District of Columbia.

The panel reviewed the center's plan for an integrated National Health Care Survey from two perspectives: (1) technical features of the plan and (2) the extent to which the survey would enable NCHS to meet the changing data needs associated with the health care policy issues discussed in the previous chapter. The following sections present the panel's review.

PERIODICITY

One feature of the center's plan is the annual data collection schedule planned for each provider survey. In recent years, primarily because of resource limitations, the average time between cycles of these surveys has increased significantly. The center correctly argues that funding and staffing these surveys on an on-again, off-again basis is not sound from a management, fiscal, or statistical point of view. It points to several advantages in fielding annual surveys, including maintaining a small group of well-trained staff, reducing the budgeting and scheduling problems associated with periodic surveys, minimizing recurrent start-up costs for survey components, addressing the seasonal nature of illness, and providing current statistics.

In order to offset the increased costs of conducting the provider surveys annually, however, the center plans to reduce their sample sizes. Reducing sample sizes obviously works against solving the general problem of producing data for subdomains of the population. The sample sizes of these surveys are too small now for subnational estimates, for estimates of diagnosis and treatment of rare conditions, and for statistics on minorities. With reduced sample size the problems of developing estimates for small areas and various subpopulations of interest appear to be aggravated.

The center plans to compensate for smaller sample sizes by aggregating data for more than one year. Although multiyear aggregation will be a necessity with the small samples, it is not clear how many years of aggregation will be necessary to produce some of the statistics needed. Furthermore, such aggregation may be less appropriate for characteristics that are not stable across years. It also will affect the timeliness of data production and analysis.

The users of data who were surveyed expressed interest in estimates below the national level, at the state level, and even at the county or community levels. The list of subpopulations of interest identified includes blacks, Hispanics, American Indians, Asians, disabled people, rural populations, specific industrial groups, elderly people, children, especially disabled children, groups defined by socioeconomic level, and people in institutions. The Disadvantaged and Minority Health Improvement Act of 1990, which contains the reauthorization of NCHS, also requires the center to develop better systems to collect data on minority subpopulations. Al-

TABLE 1 Profile of Current Survey Designs for the Three NCHS Health Provider Surveys and the National Health Interview Survey

Survey Component	National Hospital Discharge Survey (NHDS), 1988-1991	National Ambulatory Medical Care Survey (NAMCS), 1990-1991	National Nursing Home Survey (NNHS), 1994	National Health Interview Survey (NHIS), 1985-1994
Sampling design selection stage (sample size)				
1	Subsample of NHIS PSUs (112)	Subsample of NHIS PSUs (112)	Subsample of NHIS PSUs (112)	1-3 contiguous counties (198)
2	Short-stay hospitals (542: PPS with Measure of Size =Bed Size)	Office-based patient care providers (3,000: No PPS)	Long-term care providers (1,200: No PPS)	Enumeration districts/block groups
3	Inpatient discharges (250,000)	Patient visits (50,000)	Staff (4,800) Current resident (6,000) Past resident (7,200)	Area segment
Mode(s) of data collection	Records abstraction	Face-to-face (physician) Records abstraction (visit)	Face-to-face (facility) Self-administration (staff) Records abstraction (current residents) Telephone (past residents and next-of-kin)	Face-to-face

Data collected by	Bureau of the Census	Bureau of the Census	Bureau of the Census	Bureau of the Census
Frequency of data collection	Annually	Annually	Periodically (next in 1994)	Ongoing
Information needs met	Diagnosis Length of stay Procedures Discharge status	Diagnosis Source(s) of payment Duration Disposition	Facility profile Source(s) of payment Provider history Length of stay	Disability days Physician visits Acute/chronic conditions Limitation of activity Hospital stays Special topics

though not all of these expectations are realistic for national survey-based data systems, the reduced annual sample sizes planned for the National Health Care Survey will undoubtedly further aggravate the problems of developing estimates for small areas and various subpopulations at a time when NCHS is looking for ways to improve responsiveness in these areas in a cost-effective manner. The panel seriously doubts the possibility of producing small area estimates even with the proposed aggregation of data over multiple years.

The panel is informed that the NHIS sample is being redesigned to increase the sampling of PSUs in which blacks and Hispanics are concentrated. Since the National Health Care Survey will be conducted in a subsample of the NHIS PSUs, the NHIS redesign should somewhat strengthen the samples of blacks and Hispanics in the National Health Care Survey as well. However, the panel does not believe that this increase in the sampling of NHIS PSUs in which blacks and Hispanics are concentrated will improve significantly the ability of the National Health Care Survey to provide health care statistics for minority populations.

Despite the sample size deficiency, the panel believes that there are clear advantages to fielding the provider surveys on an annual basis, to reduce fluctuations in resource requirements and to ensure currency of the statistics.

Recommendation 3-1: The panel endorses the NCHS plan to conduct the components of the National Health Care Survey on an annual basis.

SCOPE AND COVERAGE

Current NCHS plans call for extending the coverage of the National Health Care Survey beyond the current four major health care provider surveys to include collection of national data for selected alternative sites of the three major types of health care and health care providers—hospital care, ambulatory care, and long-term care:

- **The Hospital and Surgical Care Component,** based on the National Hospital Discharge Survey (NHDS), is being modified to include hospital-based and free-standing ambulatory surgery centers.

- **The Ambulatory Care Component,** based on the National Ambulatory Medical Care Survey (NAMCS), is being modified to include medical care provided in emergency rooms and outpatient departments and clinics in nonfederal, short-term (i.e. average length of stay less than 30 days) hospitals. Long-range plans call for inclusion of additional settings, such as community and neighborhood health clinics.

- **The Long-Term Care Component,** based on the National Nursing Home Survey (NNHS), is being expanded to include board and care homes that provide assistance with activities of daily living, but not nursing or medical care. This addition will extend the survey to group homes, rest homes, and other supported living arrangements, including sites that provide service to the mentally and physically limited population. The long-term care component will be modified further by the inclusion of a home health care and hospices survey.

- The National Master Facility Inventory is being renamed **the National Health Provider Inventory** (NHPI) and expanded to include hospices, home health care agencies, and licensed residential care facilities. Long-range plans call for the addition of providers of acute ambulatory care and community-based long-term care to the inventory.

The panel endorses the center's efforts to extend the coverage of the provider surveys to include a range of the alternative health care settings that have emerged in recent years. The proposed extensions constitute an important step in extending the coverage of these surveys. However, they are only a first step if NCHS is to meet its responsibilities to provide a comprehensive coverage of national health care statistics in the United States.

An important further extension needed is the inclusion of services provided by nonphysicians who deliver health care. The panel's survey of users identified at least 37 types of providers and health care settings not currently being surveyed by NCHS, but for which health care statistics are needed (see Appendix B for the list of providers identified by users). Some of these health care settings are already under consideration for inclusion by NCHS. Others may not be appropriate for national surveys. Some obvious examples of additional providers for consideration are psychologists, dentists, physical and occupational therapists, pharmacists, podiatrists, chiropractors, nurses, nurse practitioners, physician assistants, nurse midwives, and optometrists, all of whom deliver some form of health care.

Another specific concern is the distinction made historically by NCHS between collection of data on the physical health services that it plans to cover, and collection of data on mental health and dental services, which are not included in the center's plan. Such a distinction seems to reflect bureaucratic issues rather than theoretical coherence. Obviously, it would not be cost-effective for NCHS to attempt to duplicate the data collection efforts of the National Institute of Mental Health, the National Institute of Dental Research, or the Health Resources and Services Administration. The panel believes, however, that NCHS should consider the collection and/or dissemination of adequate statistics about mental health and dental services to be part of its responsibility; it should furthermore ensure, perhaps through collaborative efforts, that the needed data in these areas are available from appropriate agencies and that they are collected in a form that is consistent with that used in the other provider surveys.

Finally, though ambulatory care coverage is the area most in need of expansion beyond the current plan, the hospital care component also needs to be expanded. The omission of federal hospitals and long-term care hospitals from the hospital care component is a significant deficiency. NCHS has made efforts in the past to obtain data on federal hospital discharges, and the task has proven difficult. While recognizing the difficulties, the panel nevertheless considers that it would be desirable to have integrated data on all hospitalizations, including those in federal hospitals.

Recommendation 3-2: The panel recommends that NCHS extend its coverage of providers of health care to include a fuller range of health providers than currently planned—both physicians and nonphysicians. The panel further recommends that the universe for the hospital care component be extended to include long-term care hospitals and federal hospitals.

The panel does not mean to suggest that all possible health care providers should be surveyed each year. A strategy needs to be developed for sampling types of providers at varying periodicities, with priorities based on their relative importance. For instance, periodicities for specific provider groups could be based on such considerations as expenditures for care, distribution and volume of users, political or policy issues of importance, and availability of resources. Certain categories of providers may have to be approached through periodic special studies.

At the present time, however, no objective process exists for deciding which providers should be given priority for inclusion in the surveys, except availability of resources from the parties interested in the data. A mechanism is needed for developing standard criteria for setting priorities for incorporating new and emerging settings and the full range of health care providers, as well as for periodic review and revision of these criteria as needed.

Recommendation 3-3: The panel recommends that NCHS put in place a mechanism for developing criteria and for setting data collection priorities across the full range of health care providers and service settings, and that this mechanism and process be dynamic and include periodic review and revisions of both the criteria and coverage as necessary.

DATA COLLECTED

The panel was asked to review the content of the questionnaires and definitions used in the provider surveys in terms of appropriateness and adequacy. The panel is in general agreement with the content areas included in the center's plans; however, it finds the coverage of the data content deficient in terms of what is needed to address current and future health care policy issues, as described in Chapter 2. The panel recognizes that any significant expansion or change in the data collected in the National Health Care Survey will require a major increase in the level of effort and associated resources. Nonetheless, the panel has identified several key issues that are not reflected either in the content of existing surveys or in the plan for the proposed National Health Care Survey in its current stage of development; they are discussed below.

The provider surveys that serve as the basis for the National Health Care Survey proposed by NCHS currently collect data only on events, such as individual physician visits or individual hospital discharges. Historically, NCHS has provided basic information for a broad range of issues related to the supply and volume of health care, but has lacked person-based information on health care received by individuals over time or over the entire progression of an illness episode, from onset to completion. However, policy analysts and other data users also need data on persons and about the medical care received by them in order to answer questions about episodes of illness, outcomes, costs and expenditures for care, insurance coverage, the use of multiple providers, etc. The person-based longitudinal approach would also allow for linkage to the death record through the National Death Index (NDI)[2] to obtain the mortality status of those persons being followed longitudinally. Linkage with birth records will be needed in pregnancy related to outcome studies.

The cost of health care is one of the most important health policy issues confronting the nation today. Although the NCHS statutory mandate includes monitoring health care costs and financing, including trends in health care prices and costs, the sources of payment for health services, and the federal, state, and local government expenditures for health services, it collects almost no information on payers or costs and expenditures for care (including the component paid by insurance) in a survey of health care use

---

[2]The National Death Index is a central computerized file of death record information for all deaths in the United States. It is compiled from magnetic tapes submitted to the NCHS by the state vital statistics offices. These tapes, beginning with deaths occurring in 1979, contain a standard set of identifying information for each decedent for use in searches of the NDI file to identify and locate state death records. The NDI is used by researchers conducting prospective and retrospective studies to determine if persons in their studies may have died.

(see Appendix D). The panel recognizes the difficulties in obtaining this information, but it firmly believes that a National Health Care Survey is a logical vehicle to collect data on costs and expenditures of care.

The NHDS collects information on discharges, not individuals, so data on readmissions are not available. In addition, information on the functional status of individuals would make the information on hospitalization more valuable; at the present time there is nothing on functional status in hospital discharge abstracts. The panel recognizes that the feasibility issues with respect to measuring functional status of hospitalized patients are numerous, but, if they could be overcome, research on outcomes of hospital care would be greatly strengthened. This need for more information on health and functional status of the patient for the purpose of evaluating outcomes extends, of course, to all provider sites and should be recognized in all the provider surveys.

Information on the longitudinal dimensions of care is of critical importance in order to assess the effect of treatment. Current data sets do not permit construction of meaningful patterns of care over time. This has been particularly problematic in long-term care, although there have been notable efforts to begin to correct this problem in the most recent National Nursing Home Survey. The panel is encouraged to note that some of the needed information on the residents will be available from the follow-up study to the 1985 National Nursing Home Survey. However, there is no indication in the center's plan that collection of such information will continue as part of the long-term care component of the proposed new survey.

There is need to link multiple admissions of individuals rather than treating each admission as a new patient, as is currently the case in NHDS, NAMCS, and NNHS. Such linkage would especially enhance the value of the National Nursing Home Survey. Almost one-third of all nursing home discharges are to hospitals (NCHS, 1981). Estimates suggest that one in five nursing home residents has a hospital admission each year. Research suggests that inappropriate use of the hospital by nursing home residents is a significant hidden cost of long-term care and amounts to cost shifting in a substantial proportion of cases from Medicaid to Medicare, with possible adverse health outcomes for patients (Aiken, et al., 1985; Shaughnessy,1990). Yet it has not been possible to study the patterns of care and interchange of patients between hospitals and nursing homes from the current NCHS data sets.

To be maximally useful, existing provider surveys do not include sufficient data on characteristics of providers and their practice patterns. A valuable addition would be to increase the amount of information about the various facilities, settings, and providers in which sampled events occur. For the hospitalization component, data should be collected about corporate structure, and other related variables of short-term hospitals should be added from the American Hospitalization Association's files. For ambulatory care in private offices, the kind of corporate arrangement in which physicians are practicing, the mix of specialties, the number of physicians involved in a group (if it is a group), and relationships to managed insurers constitute information that would be useful in tracking what is happening to ambulatory care.

In recent years there has been major growth in specialized units in general hospitals such as specialized psychiatric units, alcohol treatment units, and drug detoxification and treatment units. Patients treated in these units are different from those treated in "scatter" beds, and patterns of service, length of stay, and costs differ for patients in these units compared with patients with comparable diagnoses treated in general medical units. NCHS needs to develop plans to obtain information on patients seen in such special units of general hospitals. This deficiency is easily corrected by a simple coding change to indicate whether the patient was treated in a specialized unit.

An important new data collection activity that NCHS should explore is the addition of data from medical records or charts to the content of the National Health Care Survey. As mentioned previously, a major limitation, not only of NCHS surveys, but also of virtually all data sets about health care services, is the lack of detailed information on the tests and services performed during the various treatment events. The addition of such data from medical records or charts to the content of the surveys is critical to at least three important areas of research: (1) studies related to the appropriateness of care, (2) studies of outcomes and efficacy of treatments, and (3) studies of costs of treatment.

As a first step, a sample of charts from hospital discharges and from ambulatory care visits should be drawn. The information to be abstracted from these charts should be able to address issues such as:

- What tests were performed.

- Details on how patients were treated. This information is critical to outcome studies to evaluate the efficacy of alternative ways of treating patients. Details about treatments are also essential for evaluating information about the cost of care and for producing comprehensive statistics on health care use. In particular, insurance claims do not have information about noncovered services. For example, the administrative system of Medicare does not provide information about the use of prescription drugs. Moreover, providers outside the traditional fee-for-service system, such as health maintenance organizations (HMOs), typically do not file insurance claims in detail. As a result, in order to get any information about the value of delivered care, it is necessary to collect the detail that appears only on hospital and medical charts.

NCHS will play a major role in the years to come in monitoring the progress of the department's Health Objectives for the Year 2000 (U.S. DHHS, 1991a). NCHS has responsibility for tracking about 160 of more than 300 objectives. Although most of these objectives involve promotion of healthful behaviors in the population, rather than health systems performance per se, 28 specific objectives do relate to health care. Although NCHS is not currently collecting the needed information, the panel is informed that 20 of these objectives could be addressed by adding questions about physician practices to the physicians induction questionnaire for the National Ambulatory Medical Care Survey in order to assess patient treatment and health promotion activities.

NCHS should start collection of the additional information beginning with the next cycle of the National Ambulatory Medical Care Survey so that baseline data will be available to measure progress toward the department's Health Objectives for the Year 2000.

The content areas identified above are needed now and will continue to be needed in the foreseeable future, for policy analysis of the critical health care issues both for the 1990s and into the next century. It is essential therefore that NCHS move boldly into new areas of data collection and new methods that are required to obtain the needed data to meet the challenges of the next century.

Recommendation 3-4: The panel recommends that the National Health Care Survey include collection of *person-based* longitudinal information, expanding the data collected to include, but not be limited to, information on the health care received, costs and gross expenditures for health care, and outcomes.

DESIGN FEATURES

Cluster Survey Design

A central feature of the center's plan for the National Health Care Survey is to move from the existing four independently designed provider surveys to a three-stage cluster sample design[3] and to link the sample selection of these surveys geographically with the sampling design of the National Health Interview Survey (NHIS). Under this design the health care providers are to be sampled at the second stage from a first-stage sample of geographic areas, rather than selecting the providers at the first stage. The geographic areas currently being used for fielding the new survey are a

---

[3]Cluster sampling, frequently used by statisticians in designing surveys, is a method of sampling in which a population is first defined as groups or clusters of primary units and then from these groups a sample is selected.

subsample of the primary sampling units for the NHIS. This linkage with NHIS is consistent with the center's decision to base the NCHS Integrated Design Program on the NHIS sample and to establish survey linkages to the other NCHS population surveys (see Appendix A). Other features being considered by NCHS include the possible use of the same samples of health care providers over time and for several components of the National Health Care Survey in order to increase data quality and to reduce sample induction costs.

The center has identified in its plan several potential advantages: (1) increased analytic utility, since health care use is examined in relation to health status indicators from the NHIS; (2) reduced interviewing costs, since sample providers are concentrated in specific geographic areas; (3) increased potential for record linkage across settings, which aids in tracking patients and in differentiating multiple episodes of the same condition; and (4) the possibility of producing local area statistics, for sampled areas or communities.

The stated advantages of moving to a cluster sample design are being examined by NCHS. Research is currently under way for the next cycle of the NHIS redesign based on the 1990 census, including not only issues related to the NCHS population surveys, but also particular requirements of the NCHS provider surveys. Factors related to subdomain statistics, alternative design options, including the redefinition of PSUs in terms of health service areas, the effect of conducting the National Health Care Survey components in a subsample of the NHIS PSUs, and the analytical utility of such a design are being explored as part of the redesign effort. Results of this research are beginning to be available to NCHS.

In reviewing the center's proposed survey design, it becomes clear that there are two related but distinct aspects to the issue of the use of geographic areas as the primary sampling units in the cluster survey design: (1) the use of NHIS PSUs and (2) the definition of PSUs, i.e., current NHIS PSUs that are population based or PSUs defined in terms of health service areas.

Use of NHIS Primary Sampling Units

The panel believes that there may be some practical advantages to having the National Health Care Survey and the NHIS conducted in the same PSUs. It is possible that there will be efficiencies in sharing data collection staff (trained Census Bureau field staff), although the real benefits cannot be assessed until the actual strategies for data collection are fully in place. Furthermore, the assumed cost savings of having the providers geographically clustered needs to be demonstrated. The trade-off between reduced costs through use of a clustered provider sample and the impact of this design on the efficiency of the sample needs to be examined further. NCHS staff estimates suggest that, for national estimates, the loss of efficiency will be modest, less than 6 percent for the NHDS (Shimizu and Cole, 1990). The panel is not aware of similar research for the NAMCS but would be surprised if the results were worse, given the apparent correlation between physician and population geographic distributions. The panel seriously doubts the possibility of producing local area estimates by conducting the survey in a subsample of the NHIS PSUs, even with the planned multiyear aggregation of data. As stated earlier in the chapter, given the current sample sizes, the panel questions if NCHS will be able to produce reliable estimates for states, let alone for specific PSUs.

NCHS obviously has given considerable thought to the concept of an integrated National Health Care Survey and has presented arguments that its plan implies integration. The panel supports the use of the NHIS PSUs as an important first step in that direction. It should be emphasized, however, that simply conducting the provider surveys in the NHIS PSUs does not by itself result in a meaningfully integrated survey. There are a number of approaches that, taken together, would achieve greater integration with the NHIS than envisioned in the center's plan. Within the context of this survey, the panel believes that a National Health Care Survey would be considered integrated if it had the capability of obtaining relevant health care data at the person, provider, visit, or episode level that can be interlinked directly at the individual rather than at the aggregate level. Thus for example, behavioral and health status data for a sample person can be tied to such things as the use of health care facilities, the care received, the costs, and the outcome of health care received for the illness episodes that the person is experiencing.

Definition of Primary Sampling Units

The panel is skeptical about the assumption of increased analytic utility resulting from geographic linkage and by defining the PSUs in terms of health service areas. NCHS defines health service areas as one or more counties that are relatively self-contained with respect to the provision of routine hospital care. NCHS plans to be able to examine health care use in a geographic area in relation to the availability of health resources and the health status indicators from the NHIS. This would permit the computation of ecological correlations using the health service area as the unit of analysis. Recent research by Makuc and others on defining health service areas showed that, in a group of health service areas representing roughly 94 percent of the U.S. population, less than 25 percent of the hospital stays of people residing in those areas occurred outside the service area (Makuc et al., 1990). When examining patterns for ambulatory care, Kleinman and Makuc found that nearly 20 percent of physician visits occur outside the county of residence, with substantial variation according to metropolitan status, proximity to the metropolitan area, and population density (Kleinman and Makuc, 1983). No parallel research has been completed for nursing homes.

Makuc presents some examples of the kinds of analyses that could be undertaken based on the first-stage area design. Each area can be characterized by census variables and variables from other sources, such as the Area Resource File.[4] Health care data can be produced for the same areas so that such questions as the following could be answered: to what extent is one subcomponent of care being substituted for another, e.g., ambulatory surgical centers as a substitute for inpatient hospital care, hospice and home care for nursing home care? To what extent can variation in rates of utilization of health care be explained by variation in supply of providers? Small area variation in the use of health services might be used to monitor the effectiveness of the medical outcome initiatives. There are several issues that need further research before the utility of this kind of analysis can be determined. One example is the use of self-representing and non-self-representing PSUs[5] in the current National Health Interview Survey design.

Even if all the issues can be resolved, a major problem would still remain: the use of ecological correlations to draw inferences about relationships that refer to individuals. The PSUs defined in terms of health service areas may contain too diverse a population to permit valid characterization by some of the kinds of variables listed above. The internal variation may simply be too large. However, individual-level analysis can also be done by linking information about the individual health service area to the individual's health information.

In an attempt to resolve some of the issues identified above, research was undertaken by both the NCHS and the Bureau of the Census, as part of the overall NHIS redesign research, to attempt to define health service areas that would maximize the proportion of individuals receiving their health care within the defined areas, as well as to measure the effects of using these areas as PSUs on the precision of the survey estimates. The panel has learned that, on the basis of the findings of this research, NCHS has made the design decision to retain for the 1995 NHIS redesign the existing defini-

---

[4] The Area Resource File is a county-level health resources database containing over 7,000 health professions and related data elements for each county in the United States. The purpose of the file is to summarize statistics from many disparate sources into a single file in order to facilitate analysis and planning of the geographical distribution of health professionals and health resources. The Area Resource File contains data on geographic descriptor codes and classifications, health professions, health characteristics and economic data, expenditures, and environment. The data are drawn from major national surveys completed by numerous federal agencies and professional associations.

[5] A self-representing primary sampling unit is one that is included in the sample with certainty.

tion of PSUs. There is also some concern that defining PSUs in terms of health service areas increases the NHIS sampling errors, the design effects being somewhat larger for the Hispanic population. Another factor influencing the decision is the fact that the health service areas cross state boundaries, thus making the NHIS redesign less appropriate for producing state statistics. Analytic justifications for changing the PSU definition are lacking at this time. This decision does not preclude consideration of redefining the PSUs for the next NHIS redesign; in the interim, however, more research needs to be undertaken before the next NHIS redesign to determine the analytic gains, if any, and the cost consequences of redefining the NHIS PSUs.

In summary, the concept of defining a geographic area in which most of the providers serving a population are located and most of the population receiving services from the providers in that area are also located is appealing. However, there are major difficulties in defining a health service area across a range of services and different types of providers. For example, the service areas for treatment of rare or serious conditions may not coincide with the service areas for primary care. Moreover, there appears to be serious loss in efficiency in using these areas as PSUs in the sample design. The panel has not seen any definitive evidence at this time of the feasibility or analytic justification of redefining the PSUs in terms of health service areas on a national level, particularly since the health service areas can be used in analyses of NCHS surveys without using them to define PSUs. The panel, however, supports the center's intention to continue the needed research in this area.

Recommendation 3-5: The panel endorses the NCHS decision to use the primary sampling units from the National Health Interview Survey for the National Health Care Survey, to retain their existing definition at this time, and to continue the needed research in this area.

Patient Follow-up Component

The center's plan for the National Health Care Survey includes development of the capability to conduct routine and specialized patient follow-up studies of the sample event (visit, discharge, or admission) to obtain information beyond what is available in provider records. Data will be collected from the patient or the patient's family about the patient outcome, including subsequent use of medical care and morbidity, changes in health status, and quality of care. The development of the follow-up component will build on the experience gained from the 1985 National Nursing Home Survey Follow-up and the various follow-up studies of their population-based surveys. NCHS also anticipates linking these data with other data sources, just as the National Nursing Home Survey is being linked to the National Death Index to obtain mortality status information on former patients.

Discussed below are some of the potential values of the design involving follow-up of patients whose visits and discharges are sampled for the provider surveys; some of the methodological, legal, and feasibility issues that will need to be resolved before such studies can be undertaken; and the limitations of such an event-based approach to obtain the kinds of health care data needed.

There are a number of potential benefits of the planned follow-up component to the National Health Care Survey:

- Data could be collected in the follow-up component to enable patients to be characterized in terms of their health status, demographic characteristics, health behaviors, and other use of medical care.

- Data could be collected from the patient or the patient's family over a period of time about the results of treatment for the sampled event, including use of medical care and morbidity subsequent to the sampled event, changes in health status, hospital readmissions, and quality of care.

- A patient follow-up study could be conducted to focus on specific issues such as a financing mechanism; particular demographic or other groups of interest; a particular disposition at discharge; a diagnosis, condition, or procedure; or any emerging issue.

- Follow-up interviews with patients open the possibility of collecting meaningful data on gross expenditures from providers of the medical care and from insurers who paid for the service, at least for the specific sampled event.

- Patterns of care could be described for at least a subset of health care events, which could enhance the analytic value of the data about those services provided.

An important current concern in health policy research is the evaluation of the effect of various patterns of treatment and medical care on patient well-being. To address such issues, it is necessary to collect data directly from patients about their health status, symptoms, and quality of life at one or more points after they have received health care services and treatments. Once a mechanism is in place for contacting patients who are sampled in ambulatory or hospital settings; it would become possible to initiate special studies of the results of those treatments and the medical outcomes associated with those sampled events.

Unresolved Issues

One of the problems inherent in the event-based follow-up design is the need to get consent from patients for their health provider to release to NCHS the name and address information needed in order to approach the individual patients selected for follow-up. For patients whose visits were sampled in an ambulatory setting, two alternative designs present themselves: (1) ambulatory care providers could be asked ex post facto to contact the sample patients to gain permission for subsequent follow-up or to allow for their patients to be contacted directly for follow-up and (2) interviewers could interact with the patient directly in the physician's office. The latter approach is similar to the design used in the Medical Outcome Study (Tarlov et al., 1989). In that project, an interviewer was continually present in the physician's office during the sampling period. The interviewer can explain the study, obtain needed release permissions, obtain information needed for subsequent contact, and obtain data from patients. Although this procedure would obviously require feasibility testing, and certainly would constitute a major change in current survey procedures, the fact that such a design has been used by others makes it worth serious consideration. The feasibility, costs, and effectiveness of each of these procedures would need to be investigated. A field study of the cost and effectiveness of these approaches might also be considered in conjunction with any study to test feasibility of alternative procedures to obtain names and addresses of sampled patients.

Similar types of issues must be addressed for a sample of discharged patients who were in the hospitalization survey sample. Permission will be needed also from the hospital administrator to release to NCHS information about the hospitalized patient, either at the time of admission or after the discharge. One approach that can be considered is to have sampled hospitals routinely ask for a release from all patients upon admission during a sample period. An alternative approach is a passive consent procedure whereby hospitals would mail to the discharged patients notification that their names (nothing about their conditions) would be transmitted to NCHS unless patients request that they not be. Matching the patient records to interview responses would occur only after patients had been informed and had signed a consent form for the interviewer. Both approaches would require considerable effort on the part of hospital employees. The feasibility and acceptability to hospitals and patients of alternative ways to gain patient consent for follow-up need to be explored and tested. Moreover, state laws vary widely on release of information on hospitalized patients.

In addition to the issues identified above, there are several other methodological issues that need to be addressed to assess the feasibility of the event-based follow-up design, such as the efficacy of alternative ways to deal with the problem of linkage between providers, visits, and persons; the extent of attrition occurring during the process of contacting patients for follow-up through the provider setting in which they were identified (i.e., hospital or ambulatory care provider); and the problem of constructing sampling frames for providers other than those covered by existing surveys in order to conduct the follow-up studies as planned by NCHS.

Research needs to be undertaken to evaluate the feasibility and effectiveness of each of these issues and procedures, including an examination of the literature to assess how effective these procedures have been when used in previous studies.

Limitation of Event-based Follow-up Design

Although the panel supports the center's desire to develop capability for collecting data directly from patients through follow-up, a key issue in the design suggested in the plan is the appropriateness of an event-based sample for follow-up studies. *A major limitation of the National Health Care Survey as presently designed is that all the provider surveys begin with a sample of events and not persons.* That means that the probability of selection of any individual patient depends on the number and type of eligible services that he or she receives. In the ambulatory care component of the survey, for instance, people are sampled proportionate to their use of ambulatory services in physicians' offices. Although that may be a straightforward way to sample events, it is not an efficient design for producing person-based statistics. Many health conditions produce multiple visits to an ambulatory care setting; NCHS needs to determine the extent of the confounding problem resulting from the use of an event-based survey. The conceptual development of the issues involved in samples of events versus persons as a unit of analysis has lagged; there is a clear need to think about these issues in a more concrete and systematic manner than is possible within the constraints of this study. Laumann and Knoke (1987), for example, devote an extended theoretical discussion in their book *The Organizational State* to the actor-event interface and the analytic and methodological problems engendered by taking the focal analytic unit to be the actor or the event, and the need to see that these analytic units are, in fact, intimately interrelated in myriad ways. Their perspective is especially congenial to researchers who have adopted network-related analytic techniques.

Analyses of costs and outcomes depend on identifying meaningful clinical events. Some service events are meaningful units to sample. The best examples are those surgical procedures that almost always occur in hospital settings and that usually occur only once to an individual. For example, sampling hospital discharge records is a meaningful way to sample people who experience gall bladder surgery or appendectomy. Starting with such a sample, one could collect data about related services and interview patients at a later date about the complications and benefits of surgery. All hospitalizations, however, do not always produce meaningful data. For example, hospital admissions for cancer could serve as a sampling frame to describe the characteristics of those hospitalized for cancer and the services that they utilize, their costs, and how they were feeling at some later point. However, the same case of cancer could produce multiple admissions, and for some analytic purposes the omission of those who had cancer but were not hospitalized at the time (and hence were not represented in the statistics) could constitute a serious problem.

In summary, the follow-up design described by NCHS potentially adds to the value of the data collected from the NHDS and the NAMCS for studying certain conditions. NCHS has made a case for sampling clinically meaningful events from provider-based samples. Treatments that usually occur only once constitute one class of health care that can be studied from such samples. Health conditions that almost invariably lead an individual to seek care from a provider, such as a broken hip, a broken leg, or a heart attack, also probably can be meaningfully sampled from event-based sample frames. There are real practical problems, however, associated with obtaining permission and contacting a high percentage of sampled patients. There are multiplicity problems associated with sampling to be resolved, arising from the fact that an individual's chance of selection depends on the number of health care events the individual had for the condition (Sirken, 1972a, 1972b; Nathan, 1976).

CONCLUSION

The panel supports the center's primary objective for the National Health Care Survey. The panel is concerned, however, that, as currently designed, the survey appears to be limited mostly to modest modifications and coverage extensions of the existing provider-based surveys, with minimal, if any, true integration of design and data. Yet the concept of a National Health Care Survey is a broad and challenging concept. If the center's objective, as stated in its plan, is to move in the direction of an integrated survey design to provide comprehensive health care data that are urgently needed, especially on access, expenditures, disease episodes, and outcomes, then such an objective should have a major impact on the design and content of their surveys. NCHS cannot get that kind of statistical information from a sample of events, which is its current approach.

Although NCHS provider surveys have considerable strengths in measuring the health services provided in traditional medical care settings and in some alternative care settings in the near future, they reflect only part of the care provided in the United States today. Each of the NCHS provider surveys on health care is oriented toward providing data on services received for the sampled event in the respective facility. When taken together, they do not represent a comprehensive approach to the collection of the needed data on the nation's health care system.

NCHS has proposed strategies to address some of the gaps in the data from its existing provider-based surveys. The panel supports these initiatives; however, the panel believes that the center's vision for a National Health Care Survey falls short of a plan for meeting anticipated health care information needs today and into the next century, even with the suggestions contained in this chapter for changes and improvements. The panel strongly urges the center to become more comprehensive in its approach to meeting the data needs identified in this report. A strategy that is flexible enough to adapt to changes and new fast-breaking directions requires a more integrated and a more visionary course of action than currently planned by NCHS. The next chapter provides the panel's recommendations for a design framework that would lead to a more integrated National Health Care Data System that will provide the basis for such a flexible, long-term data collection and implementation strategy.

4

Design for a National Health Care Data System

The foregoing discussion makes it clear that the panel believes that existing data systems are not adequate to yield the range of statistical information needed to fully address the complex health care issues facing this nation. NCHS has proposed a general strategy to expand and extend its provider-based surveys to be more responsive to data needs and has taken the first steps toward geographically integrating them with the National Health Interview Survey (NHIS). These proposed changes, however, do not satisfy the urgent needs for data to monitor the health care of the nation.

The panel's appraisal has demonstrated that, as currently conceived, the center's plan does not provide the capacity to address important questions about the interrelationships between the health status of individuals and the patterns and cost of health care services they receive from a broad range of providers and service settings over time. The long-term agenda, therefore, requires consideration of further, more fundamental restructuring.

Since a design is dictated by the objectives of a data system, this chapter first briefly states the panel's perception of the objectives of a National Health Care Data System and then presents the panel's recommended design framework for achieving these objectives. The benefits and limitations of the proposal are discussed, and issues that require further research are identified in the discussion. The chapter concludes with a suggested implementation schedule.

STATEMENT OF OBJECTIVES

The objectives of the National Health Care Survey proposed by NCHS should be driven by the goals and objectives of the nation's health care system, a primary goal of which is to deliver health care services effectively and efficiently to the entire U.S. population. A simple statement then of the objectives of a National Health Care Survey would be to provide statistics on a continuing basis that reflect the condition of health care in the United States, particularly with respect to the critical issues of access, quality, and cost. Such a survey should have the capability of obtaining data related to the characteristics and health status of individuals and their demand for, and use of, health care over time and across a broad range of providers and service settings that can be linked at the individual rather than the aggregate level. Data are needed to support analysis along each of the following dimensions:

Access: there is need for information on the supply of health care providers (including information on numbers, distribution, and type) and the demand for and utilization of health care services by specific segments of the population (e.g., racial and ethnic minorities, migrant populations, the uninsured, the elderly, the disabled) and by other characteristics such as health care insurance coverage status.

Quality: there is need for information concerning the health and functional status of the patient prior to and after treatment, the appropriateness of treatments or procedures provided, the degree to which health care providers resolve problems, and the satisfaction of the patient with the process.

Cost: there is need for information on expenditures for health care services by type of provider, the cost of treatment for an episode of illness for a specific diagnosis, its distribution among provider types, and the source of payment for care provided, including how much is paid by insurance and how much is paid out-of-pocket.

In addition to obtaining information from providers, information is needed about health care consumers. For example, if a consumer has had contact with several provider types for a given episode of illness, some way has to be found to obtain that information in a coordinated way. Some people may have had no contacts with the health care system at all; this group is important to identify, and information is needed on their health care needs. For example, answers are needed to the following questions concerning the health care of consumers:

- What is their health status, in terms of disability, functional status, and chronic conditions?
- What are their unmet health care needs? What are the individual's perceptions regarding access to health care?
- What is the person's health insurance coverage, including no coverage at all?
- What is the person's use of health care providers over a defined period of time? For each episode of care? For what conditions? At what cost, both out-of-pocket and covered by insurance?
- What are the person's knowledge, attitude, and practices related to health promotion and disease prevention, such as knowledge of risk factors, attitudes toward risks, and risk behavior?
- What are the person's demographic characteristics?

No one single survey can provide answers to all these questions. An integrated data system is needed with linkage capability at the individual level that includes a variety of approaches, including surveys of specific provider types and service settings, follow-up of patients seen for specific conditions by specific types of providers in specific settings, longitudinal surveys of the household and nursing home populations, and possibly surveys of episodes of illness.

In addition, there is need for improved collaboration, coordination, and integration of health care data collected by NCHS and other agencies of the Department of Health and Human Services. Care should be taken to ensure that health care surveys carried out by NCHS and the other agencies use standard definitions and classifications and do not unnecessarily duplicate information and that other needed steps are taken to facilitate integration of data sets for analysis and dissemination.[1]

DESIGN CONSIDERATIONS

The panel was guided by three basic considerations in proposing a design framework for a National Health Care Data System:

(1) Any design proposed has to meet existing information needs, especially those currently not being met, such as those identified in Chapter 2.

---

[1]Some of the methodological issues associated with accessing, linking, and integrating data sets are discussed in Wachter and Straf (1990).

(2) As the nation's health care system changes, so too will the information needs that give the system direction. The design for the National Health Care Data System must therefore possess sufficient flexibility to be capable of responding in a timely manner to changing information needs. This flexibility should include the capability to use special supplements to ongoing surveys to quickly provide data in support of emerging information needs and to support the conduct of ad hoc special studies.

(3) The design proposed should minimize any disruption to the current NCHS survey program to facilitate implementation of any operational changes for NCHS that the design might require and, as far as possible, preserve continuity between existing and new data outputs.

A FRAMEWORK FOR A NATIONAL HEALTH CARE DATA SYSTEM

With the above design considerations driving its thinking, the panel has proposed a design strategy to meet the various data needs that have been identified in its deliberations. Some of the currently unmet needs relate to cost of care for patterns of illness, outcomes, and patterns of provider utilization during an illness, access to provider care, functional status, severity of illness prior to and after treatment, insurance coverage, information about specific population subgroups (e.g., racial and ethnic minorities, migrant populations, the uninsured, the elderly, the disabled), as well about other categories (such as providers not currently covered by NCHS provider surveys and rare illnesses).

As stated in the preceding chapter, the event-based follow-up design proposed by NCHS, as an extension of existing NCHS provider surveys, would allow NCHS to expand its provider-based data gathering to include outcomes of hospital and private practice physician care, two important and currently unmet data needs. There are major issues, however, surrounding feasibility, operating procedures, and informed consent that need to be resolved before the design could be implemented.

Certain important data needs remain unmet with the adoption of the event-based follow-up design. Some examples are the ability to produce person-based estimates of illness, access to care, patterns of care for episodes of illness, and associated costs. Still needed, therefore, is a broader strategy that addresses these unmet data needs in an effective manner.

Such a strategy is presented below, not so much as one specific design but as a design framework for a National Health Care Data System within which a variety of survey approaches linked to the NHIS can be developed, and from which a broad range of health-related information needs can be met. The panel believes that, taken as a totality, its recommended course of action represents the long-term direction in which the National Health Care Data System should evolve.

Although NCHS has taken the first important steps to expand on the coverage and content of the provider surveys and geographically linking the provider surveys with the National Health Interview Survey sample design, in the panel's judgment the NCHS has not gone far enough. The panel proposes in this chapter a comprehensive approach for the National Health Care Data System that goes beyond the expansion planned by NCHS and that links the design and operation of the National Health Interview Survey with the provider surveys. Such a strategy would provide not only new data but also a basis for linkage of data on a population-based sample of individuals with data on their health care providers, thus further enhancing the benefits.

Since a central feature of the panel's proposed design framework is to link the NHIS design with the operations of the National Health Care Data System, it is useful to review some of the design features of the existing provider surveys to see what degree of integration may already exist. As shown in Table 1 in Chapter 3, the primary sampling units for the National Hospital Discharge Survey (NHDS) and the National Ambulatory Medical Care Survey (NAMCS) are subsamples of the NHIS primary sample. This design implies that samples of providers for these two surveys are currently being chosen exclusively from lists of hospitals and medical practices that are located in some of the same areas in which NHIS interviewing is being conducted. This geographic integration, in turn, must also imply that some degree of operational coordination already exists, or should exist, among these surveys. Moreover, data collection in all these surveys is being conducted by the Bureau of the Census. Extension of this level of design integration to nursing homes is currently being planned for the next round of the National Nursing Home Survey (NNHS).

The key elements or components of the proposed framework are to:

(1) Change the origin of the provider samples from listings of providers and service settings maintained by NCHS to identification of providers and service settings by respondents to the National Health Interview Survey (at least for those providers not in the inventories maintained by NCHS).

(2) Sample from NHIS respondents to gather longitudinal person-based data on the health status and health care received by individuals along with the associated costs and expenditures.

(3) Modify the sampling design of the National Nursing Home Survey to collect longitudinal data on health care utilization by the institutionalized population not presently covered by the NHIS.

(4) Sample from NHIS respondents and collect longitudinal data on the process of health care, the utilization of providers, and the costs and expenditures associated with episodes of illness.

NHIS-Based Sampling of Providers

As discussed in Chapter 3, one of the features of the NCHS plan is to extend the types of providers to include alternative sites of health care covering hospital and surgical care, ambulatory care, and long-term care. The panel is concerned that current NCHS plans for expanding the coverage of the National Health Care Survey are not as broadly based as they should be with respect to national statistics on providers of health care. The panel therefore proposes a method for extending the coverage of providers of health care that is capable of covering the full range of providers, both physicians and nonphysicians.

Although well-developed lists of short-term hospitals, office-based physicians, and nursing homes do currently exist, a major problem with the proposed extension of health care providers is the lack of adequate lists from which these "other providers" can be sampled and the high cost of developing and maintaining up-to-date inventories for each category of health facility or provider in a set of first-stage sampling units. This section outlines the panel's proposal for a sample design that will meet in a cost-effective manner the need established by NCHS to expand its data gathering to be able to include a fuller range of providers and health care settings than currently planned.

Rather than develop separate sampling frames for each and every type of "other provider" (i.e., other than short-stay hospitals, office-based physicians, and nursing homes), the panel proposes that appropriate national samples of "other provider" categories be identified by screening National Health Interview Survey respondents for the names and addresses of the health care providers and settings they visited in a very recent period, such as a defined two-week reference period.

The essence of the proposed design is the identification by NHIS respondents of providers to be sampled for the expanded National Health Care Data System. The design is flexible, in that it can be applied for any type of provider, and it can be readily applied to collect data for new health care settings that emerge over the course of time. Each sampled provider is subsequently contacted and asked to provide data for the visit that led to the provider's selection and for a sample of other visits. Apart from the manner in which the providers are sampled, the survey procedures can be similar to those used in the current provider surveys. The basic sample design and data-gathering plan for the NHIS does not change, except that the questionnaire would have to be expanded to collect information to identify and locate providers that the respondents visited in the specified reference period.

The primary advantage of changing the origin of a sample of "other providers" from provider lists to reports of health provider care received by NHIS respondents is the significant savings in both cost and time to acquire sampling frames for each type of "other provider." The time factor is of considerable concern, particularly in a changing environment, with newly emerging modes and numbers of health care providers. The NHIS-based approach offers rapid identification of emerging health care providers, which is just not possible with the current approach of developing and maintaining inventories for given types of providers to serve as sampling frames.

Another important and attractive feature of this sample design is that the health providers in the NHIS-based sample are selected with probabilities directly proportional to their use or size (i.e., number of visits for health care they receive in a given period), provided that (a) the NHIS interviews are spread evenly throughout the time period and (b) the NHIS respondents are sampled with equal probability. In practice, the latter condition is not satisfied because, for instance, of the oversampling of minority populations. However, a subsample of NHIS respondents can be drawn in a manner that creates an equal probability sample of NHIS respondents for use in sampling providers.

The selection of providers with probabilities proportional to size (PPS) enhances the potential for increased reliability of the estimates derived from the sample of visits subsequently selected to gather utilization data from each type of provider surveyed. The selection of a constant number of visits from each selected provider yields an equal probability sample of visits and balances the data-gathering workload. Thus, for example, 20 visits might be sampled from each selected provider. The choice of the number of visits to select from each provider depends on cost and variance considerations. This number may well vary among different types of providers. Research is needed to determine the most appropriate number of visits to select from each provider.

The panel recognizes that there are a number of potential difficulties in the implementation of this design. It relies on complete reporting of visits by NHIS respondents; significant underreporting of certain types of visits (such as those for less socially acceptable diseases) could create serious problems. Also, the NHIS respondents may not be able to provide sufficiently accurate information to enable the sampled providers to be located. Some of the named providers might be located outside the NHIS PSUs, thereby increasing the cost of subsequent data collection. The sampled providers may be reluctant to provide the requested visit data. How should providers sampled in this way be approached to maximize their cooperation? Methodological studies will clearly need to be conducted on such issues before this design is implemented.

Since, for some types of provider visits, recalling visits could be problematic, the decision to limit recall to 1-2 weeks may be necessary. The only recent comparable experience on obtaining permission to contact providers from household samples comes from the National Medical Expenditure Survey (NMES), wherein signed respondent permission and successful contact were achieved for 81 percent of identified providers. Based on preliminary estimates, approximately 40 percent of the nonresponding providers in this process were lost because of an inability of the interviewer to obtain sufficient identifying information for the provider (Harper et al., 1991). The remainder were lost because of the interviewer's inability to obtain signed permission or because the provider refused to comply with the request for records data. There is also the issue of people making multiple visits to providers for different conditions and the problem of matching respondent reports to provider records. Further research would be needed to investigate the level of recall error and to minimize this attrition. Experience would suggest that keeping attrition at an acceptable level is at least possible, given the relatively high household survey response rates achieved by the NHIS.

Identifying a provider sample through a household sample chosen within well-defined primary sampling units presents the logistical problem that some providers will be located outside their boundaries, some perhaps some distance away. Since excluding providers outside the PSUs would destroy the validity of the provider sample, there is no recourse but to attempt to enroll them all. This then raises the issue of what percentage of sample providers will be located outside the boundaries and how best one might handle dealing with them. Recent experience from NMES suggests that this would be a relatively minor problem for the hospitalization and the ambulatory care components. Research would be needed, however, to find creative yet practical ways to administer these surveys for providers outside the PSU, for whom field staff might have to commute some distance.

Recommendation 4-1: The panel recommends that providers other than those currently covered—i.e., short-term hospitals, office-based physicians, and nursing homes—be surveyed using provider samples generated from the list of providers visited by respondents to the National Health Interview Survey as identified through the survey screening.

The proposed NHIS-based sample design for providers is particularly useful for providers for whom no list frames exist, and especially for newly emerging health care settings. In principle, the design could be expanded to include visits reported by NHIS respondents to short-stay hospitals and office-based physicians. Currently, since provider utilization in terms of number of visits is not known in general, the NHDS uses proxy measures of size (e.g., the number of beds) to select samples. The NAMCS is not a PPS sample, whereas the NHIS-based sample is. Thus the NHIS respondent-generated samples of short-stay hospitals and office-based physicians conceivably could be more efficient statistically. By contrast, hospitalizations (or other visits) that lead to deaths or institutionalizations will not be represented in the NHIS-based sample, with resulting biased estimation.

Clearly, many factors can enter into a decision whether or not to change the origin of the samples of short-stay hospitals and office-based physicians from inventories currently maintained by NCHS to identification of such providers by NHIS respondents. As there is insufficient information on the relative feasibility, costs, and efficiency of these alternative approaches, NCHS should research the issues prior to any final decision.

Recommendation 4-2: The panel recommends that NCHS examine the feasibility and utility of selecting its samples of short-term hospitals and office-based physicians from inventories of each of these types of providers visited by respondents to the National Health Interview Survey and identified through the survey screening.

NHIS-Based Surveying of Cohorts of Individuals

As discussed in Chapter 2, comprehensive data on the use of health care services are urgently needed on a continuous basis if the critical issues of cost, access, and quality of care are to be meaningfully addressed. This implies continuously gathering longitudinal, person-level data reflecting patterns of care sought and received, including what services were provided, by whom, and with what outcome, as well as the associated charges by type of service and how the charges were paid.

The panel believes that the National Health Care Data System can and should meet these data needs. Specifically, the panel proposes a prospective design in which the NHIS will be used to identify cohorts of individuals to be interviewed periodically over specified time periods to provide longitudinal data on their health care utilization and expenditures.[2] The national health care statistics on key policy-related items generated by these cohort surveys should be published annually.

The cohorts based on subsamples of NHIS respondents should be selected so as to permit provision of national statistics that would best address health care policy issues. In addition, oversampling should be used to sample policy-relevant cohorts such as low-income people, uninsured people, minorities, people with poor perceived health status, disabled people,

---

[2] The analysis of longitudinal data is an active area of research with many new techniques. For an introduction of this literature see Kasprzyk et al. (1989); Cox and Cohen (1985); Duncan and Kalton (1987); Heckman and Singer (1985); Kalton et al. (1989); Kasprzyk and Jacobs (1991); Office of Management and Budget (1986); Pearson (1989); Ruggles (1991).

and elderly people. Since unbiased national estimates for the general population should be generated in any event, sample cohorts representing those individuals not eligible for any of the special interest cohorts should also be selected from among the NHIS respondents and interviewed periodically as well.

To ensure the completeness and accuracy of the information reported in the follow-up interviews by sample persons on the health care services they received, the cost of those services, and the sources of payment, the providers of those services and the health insurers will need to be contacted to obtain the details of each provider visit experienced by at least a subsample of the persons in the cohort. Signed permission to make these contacts and to release the relevant data will need to be obtained from each person sampled. The relative feasibility of collecting such signed permission forms by mail versus face-to-face, for those interviewed by telephone, will need to be explored by NCHS.

Numerous design issues will need to be addressed, for example: (1) timing in the selection of the samples of NHIS respondents relative to the initiation of data collection, (2) frequency of the periodic follow-up interviews, (3) mode of the initial follow-up and repeat interviews, and (4) respondent motivation and sample attrition.

One problem that arises in selecting the samples for follow-up from NHIS respondents is the potential for a sizable time interval between the NHIS interviews and the initiation of the follow-up interviews and the attendant loss of sampled individuals who have moved in the interval. To minimize recall errors, the follow-up interviews should be conducted frequently, say once a quarter, or even more frequently if suggested by the findings of the 1987 NMES, conducted by the Agency for Health Care Policy and Research. The cost of carrying out the follow-up interviews could be mitigated by the use of computer-assisted telephone interviews whenever possible. Retention of sampled individuals for the full set of follow-up interviews is always a challenge; appropriate incentives to minimize attrition should be devised.

The selection of a sample of individuals from NHIS respondents to collect data on health care use and expenditures is not a new concept. An NCHS-funded study (Cox et al., 1987) evaluated alternative designs for linking the 1987 NMES with the NHIS. Included in the alternatives examined were optimally allocated designs that utilized data collected in the NHIS with respect to race, poverty status, age, and health status to construct strata. The study found, for example, that the NHIS-linked, optimally allocated, not-self-weighting designs for these policy-relevant strata, at least, could achieve significant cost savings for estimates of average annual utilization and expenditures by type of provider relative to the cost of achieving the precision of an unlinked design. The optimally allocated design essentially uses characteristics of NHIS respondents to oversample potentially heavy users of health care services, thereby yielding greater efficiency. This design, however, was not in the final plan for the NMES that was developed.

The panel recognizes that surveys for gathering information on medical expenditures are expensive. Yet it believes that it is important in today's environment to be informed on a current basis about health care needs, patterns of care received, and the associated costs. Linking the cohort samples to the NHIS and oversampling these samples in policy-relevant domains, together with greater use of telephone interviewing, might produce the needed data at somewhat less cost than has been experienced to date in previous population-based medical expenditure surveys.

It should be noted that the proposed design for a continuing longitudinal survey of health care utilization and expenditures is in many ways similar to that for the NMES. When fully operational this survey would gather basic data similar to the data gathered in NMES, but at a somewhat lower cost. The proposed design will use a cohort of individuals selected from the NHIS respondents, and the screening to identify providers will be done within the context of NHIS, an ongoing survey with an existing cadre of interviewers. Basic data on health care costs and expenditures (both out-of-pocket and total expenditures) will therefore be available on a more current and resource-efficient basis than is possible now from ad hoc comprehensive surveys conducted at infrequent intervals.

Recommendation 4-3: The panel recommends that NCHS develop and implement, as a component of the National Health Care Data System, a continuous, longitudinal survey of health care utilization and expenditures and their health care providers, using cohorts of individuals selected from among National Health Interview Survey respondents.

The panel believes that it is essential that NCHS work in coordination with the Agency for Health Care Policy and Research in implementing this recommendation, which it sees as a natural next step in the development of routine collection of health care cost data.

NNHS-Based Surveying of Cohorts of Residents

Currently little or no data are available for residents of nursing homes on their use and expenditures for health care services from other providers (i.e., other than the nursing home) while institutionalized. This deficiency can be addressed by collecting health care utilization and expenditures data for a sample of nursing home residents on a continuous basis in a manner comparable to that outlined in the proposed NHIS-based cohort survey. Thus a sample of current residents in each NNHS sample facility could be selected periodically, to serve as a cohort of institutionalized persons. Longitudinal data, analogous to that collected from the NHIS-based cohorts, on the use of other health providers by members of the cohort could then be collected periodically, over the course of a year, from nursing home records and from the health care providers who treated them. The field work for such a design is facilitated by the center's plan to conduct the next NNHS in the subsample of the NHIS PSUs.

The panel urges NCHS to explore the use of this method to collect health care use and expenditure data for people in other types of long-term health care institutions as well, such as mental hospitals.

Recommendation 4-4: The panel recommends that NCHS develop and implement a survey capability to obtain longitudinal data for cohorts of residents of nursing homes, while institutionalized, on their use of and expenditures for health care received from providers other than the nursing home itself. NCHS should explore the possibility of obtaining this information for residents of other long-term institutions.

There are other subgroups of the population, such as the homeless, migrant workers, people in jails and prisons, who are not well captured by the current NHIS sampling design, even when it is supplemented by nursing homes and possibly federal and long-term hospitals. The implications of excluding these groups in surveys monitoring the nations's health status and the use and costs of health services are obvious, considering that these groups are at high risk of poor health. The panel regards the appropriate representation of these subgroups, while difficult, to be very important and urges NCHS to initiate research to find ways to adequately capture these groups in their surveys.

NHIS-NNHS-Based Surveying of Episodes of Illness

An important feature of the proposed National Health Care Data System is the capability of collecting longitudinal data on the health status and health care utilization of a population-based sample of individuals and linking them with the associated information on the health care providers. The design strategy recommended in the previous sections represents a major step forward by linking information on the individuals with visits to health care providers, thus enabling important policy-related data on the condition of the health care system to be collected and reported continuously. However, the design does not necessarily capture the complete dynamics of the illness and treatment process. In order to more fully portray the health care system, data are needed that reflect the illness and treatment process from onset of the illness, diagnosis, treatment, and outcome.

Although there are a number of potential ways in which such longitudinal data on individuals can be organized (for instance, by period of observation), an attractive organizational concept from many standpoints is the "episode of illness" and the patterns of care associated with such episodes. The episode model focuses on the observed patterns of care as a reflection of the care sought and received in conjunction with an episode of illness through possible treatment and outcome. Thus an alternative approach to gathering population-based statistics on health care services, wherein one follows a cohort of individuals, could be to limit the longitudinal data collection to those persons reporting an illness episode. This model could be used for studying patterns of utilization, cost of care, quality and access to care, and the role of the different types of providers and technologies. Since only those persons experiencing an episode of illness would be followed, this approach also has the potential to gather the requisite health care data more efficiently than from a cohort representing all persons, as presented earlier, and could conceivably replace it in the long run.

The panel recognizes that despite the attractiveness of the concept and its many advantages, its application has been relatively limited because of practical difficulties. Steinwachs (1991) identifies several problem areas that have limited the use of the episode of illness concept in examining health services utilization. These include the lack of standard definitions and classifications to be used in constructing the episode of care resulting from an episode of illness, as well as the lack of standard summary measures of episode characteristics, such as duration of an episode, intensity of care, level of use, cost, and outcomes.[3] The application of the episode concept to chronic conditions is not clear: Is there a single long episode, or is it more properly conceptualized as a series of episodes for maintenance, care, or treatment of acute exacerbations?

These issues should be resolvable, both from methodological and resource perspectives. In particular, classifications will need to be developed to resolve such issues as: When does an episode begin (e.g., does it require limitation in activity for at least one day)? When does an episode of illness end (e.g., is this the last day of any limitation)? When does the care for the illness end, how should comorbidities be identified and included in the episode, when is the episode part of a chronic disease process and when is an acute and time limited condition, and when should outcomes be measured (e.g., single or multiple points in time)? Clearly, an investment in methodological work is needed by NCHS and the Agency for Health Care Policy and Research to resolve these and other issues before pursuing the theoretical attractiveness of the episode concept into application, particularly in large-scale surveys.

---

[3]Recent literature examining definitional and operational issues associated with episode of care analysis includes, among others, Keeler (1991, 1988a, 1988b), Hornbrook (1985), Starfield et al. (1991), Frank et al. (1991), and Prien et al. (1991).

Assuming that the definitional and related issues are resolved, the panel proposes a design that would efficiently use survey resources to develop episode information. Within the context of a population survey, those individuals reporting a recent onset of an episode of illness (within two weeks) would be the target population, including mental and emotional illnesses. This group can be expected to include many minor self-limited illnesses or injuries for which no care is sought, yet there may be some individuals who are at the early stage of a serious condition and have not received care or made an appointment for care. It would be important to follow all individuals seeking care, plus those who have not sought care, to the end of the episode of illness or to the end of the care process, which ever comes later. This would provide unique information on patient outcomes, their relationship to care seeking and to the pattern of care received from one or more providers. The interpretation of the interview and follow-up data can be substantially enhanced by supplementing these data with information from providers and patient records for those episodes receiving care.

The population can be viewed as consisting of people with different patterns of illness. For example, experience would range from no episodes during the specified reference period through minor episodes of relatively short duration, that require no provider care, to acute episodes that would require provider care and end in either death or recovery. Some individuals may experience more than one illness episode (possibly overlapping) during the period. The majority of persons with short-duration episodes would be part of the noninstitutionalized portion of the population. More episodes associated with chronic conditions (i.e., those extending over longer periods of time) than short-term acute episodes are often experienced by persons institutionalized in long-term health care facilities.

A sample of eligible individuals with selected episodes would be followed until the outcome of the episode occurs, or until some operationally defined stopping point is reached (e.g., six months after onset, some defined state of health or disability). Defining a stopping point for episodes such as injuries with a permanent disability is complicated, even if an arbitrary time period after onset is used. A full range of data (e.g., diagnosis, provider visits, costs and treatment strategies tied to individual provider visits, limitation of activities, and final outcome) would be gathered for each selected episode from health care providers and insurers.

Identifying information about each reported provider, along with signed permission to abstract data from the medical and accounting records for the respondent at each identified provider, would be obtained at the conclusion of each initial and each follow-up interview. Permission forms for the providers visited at the time of the first interview may not be sufficient, since persons may go to other providers after that time. The length of the reference period must reflect the respondent's ability to recall visits and minor episodes.

The episode of illness model illustrated here is linked to the NHIS design and operation. Except for expansion to the NHIS questionnaire to accommodate screening for illness episodes in addition to obtaining identifying information for visited providers from the list of providers, the existing design and data gathering plan for the NHIS would not change. The process of screening is similar to that described for the other components of the design framework described in the preceding sections and would proceed in the manner described below.

The NHIS respondents first would be screened to determine those who began an episode of illness during a short reference period immediately prior to the interview. Thus, a representative sample of the group of illness episodes occurring to individuals over a time period of interest would be defined, then repeat contacts would be made to chart the course of the episode and to determine when it was completed. Contacts would be made with the providers of care for the episode to collect data on the treatment process, outcome, and costs.

A subsample of the NHIS respondents would be screened for all providers visited and illness episodes suffered during a recent reference period. Two types of illness episodes can be identified through this screening process: (1) those with one or more provider visits (other than to NNHS-eligible nursing homes) occurring during some reference period ending just prior to the regular NHIS interview and (2) those that ended during the same reference period but for which no provider visits occurred during the course of the episode (e.g., colds, flu, minor injury, and illness for which one cannot afford to seek care). Only those persons experiencing a "new" illness episode that led to utilization of medical care would be eligible for follow-up. In other words, the subset of illness episodes, with a provider visit occurring during the reference period, becomes the sampling frame of illness episodes screened for further follow-up beyond the NHIS screening interview. By restricting the sample to episodes that begin in the two-week period immediately prior to interview, the sampling probabilities for the group of episodes are easily determined and the complication of selecting episodes with probabilities proportional to their length is avoided.

A major limitation of this model as illustrated is that the emphasis on new episodes does not adequately address the need for information on chronic illness care, both routine maintenance and acute problems. An option for capturing information on the treatment of chronic conditions is to determine if during the past two weeks the individual experienced limitations in activity related to a chronic condition. If yes, information could be sought regarding whether the limitation was more severe, the same, or less severe than previously. If the limitation is worse, this would define a "new" episode in the ongoing care of the chronic condition. These would be followed using a methodology parallel to episodes for conditions that are not identified as chronic.

It is also likely that a significant number of people experiencing a chronic condition will never experience a well-defined "chronic episode," with a well-defined beginning and end, yet will interact with health care providers periodically. If that is the case, use of the episode of illness approach would be limited to episodes of acute illness. Under such circumstances, a sample of NHIS respondents with chronic conditions would need to be identified and interviewed periodically to determine their utilization and expenditures for health care during a time period of interest, such as a calendar year.

Since residents of nursing homes (or other long-term care institutions) are not included in the NHIS, selection of a subsample of current residents of the NNHS sample facilities should be considered for tracking episodes of illness that require health care services to be sought outside the nursing home. To facilitate episode screening, the NNHS sample would be subsampled, similar to the NHIS household sample. To properly reflect seasonal variations in illnesses, the NNHS subsample should be evenly spread over time.

The episode screening of sampled nursing home residents would be carried out in similar fashion to the screening of the NHIS respondent subsample. The purpose of the screening is to identify any episode that led to medical care during the reference period, not including the episode that caused the sampled individual to become a patient in the nursing home. The information to be collected for residents suffering an episode of illness should be essentially the same as that collected about episodes of illness occurring to the NHIS respondent subsample.

Recommendation 4-5: The panel recommends that NCHS undertake research in collaboration with the Agency for Health Care Policy and Research to examine the methodological issues of definitions and classifications and to determine the feasibility of using the National Health Interview Survey and the National Nursing Home Survey to generate a sample of episodes of illness; the sample should be followed longitudinally to collect data on the associated medical care use for the episode from both the sample of individuals and the health care providers.

Effectiveness and Efficiency

In the face of rapidly rising health care costs, there is growing interest in treatment effectiveness in relation to cost. The episode of illness model offers an opportunity to collect not only data on each component of health care received and their costs, but also data on the outcomes of that care. Broadly based national statistics bearing on the overall effectiveness and efficiency of the U.S. health care system would thus become possible.

The validity and cost of gathering health care data from health care consumers suggest that every effort should be made to take advantage of administrative records, such as health insurance claims files from both private and public insurers, patient medical records, and patient billing records. Medicare claims files provide a unique opportunity to study health care services received and costs for Medicare recipients. A similar set of claims files is needed for a national sample of persons younger than age 65.

Recommendation 4-6: The panel recommends that NCHS conduct research and develop procedures for data systems that enable linkage of health care outcomes to health care received and health care costs. The panel further urges NCHS to examine the feasibility of collecting health insurance claims files from both private and public insurers for individuals included in the samples selected from the National Health Interview Survey and the National Nursing Home Survey to study health care utilization and costs.

Relation to the NHIS Redesign

As stated early in the chapter, a central feature of the panel's recommendations is to link the NHIS design to the operations of the National Health Care Data System. Work is under way on the 1995 redesign of the NHIS based on the 1990 decennial census, which will affect NHIS data collection for at least 10 years. The decisions made on the NHIS redesign will therefore have implications for the successful and timely implementation of the panel's recommendations for an integrated design framework for collecting health care data.

Recommendation 4-7: The panel recommends that NCHS take into serious consideration the recommendations in this report relating to the National Health Care Data System before reaching final decisions on the 1995 redesign of the National Health Interview Survey.

POTENTIAL BENEFITS OF THE PROPOSED DESIGN FRAMEWORK

Adopting the panel's recommended design framework for a National Health Care Data System has several potential advantages, some of which

TABLE 2   Summary of Data Produced Under the Design Framework

Level	Linked to NHIS Through	Data Collected Under Design Framework[a]
Person	NHIS respondent	Disability days Physician visits Acute/chronic conditions Limitations of activities Hospital stays Insurance coverage Special topics *Access to care* *Preventive care*
Episode[b]	First provider visit during an episode	*Cost of care* *Episode outcome* *Pattern of provider care* *Incidence/prevalence* *Duration* *Content of provider care* *Severity of illness* *Access to care*
Visit	Any provider visit during episode	Diagnosis Length of stay Disposition Treatment *Cost of care*
Provider	Any provider visit whether or not for an episode	Facility profile *Health promotion practices* *Treatment practices*

[a]Currently unmet needs in italics.
[b]Includes only illness episodes leading to the utilization of health care. Minor episodes not requiring provider visits are also reported by respondents to the National Health Interview Survey.

are tied to meeting unmet information needs (Table 2). The data system when fully implemented would produce substantial new data at the person and visit level. Some of the new items are simply add-ons to questionnaires for the existing provider surveys; others would be obtained from new survey activities. The proposed data system in the long run would also provide a unique population-based database to facilitate assessment of the cost-effectiveness of treatment programs for specific health conditions.

The panel's proposed data system would be able to meet the need for direct data linkage between the person and provider data. Information gathered for any treatment event, including data on providers visited or individual provider visits, can be linked to the person who reported the provider and the visit. Thus, for example, data on the condition for which the treatment was provided and its outcome could be related to the socioeconomic characteristics of the individual. Linkage between person-level and provider-level data also provides a basis for confirming the illness diagnosis.

The proposed data system would give NCHS sufficient flexibility to be able to adapt to changing data needs. One important facet of this flexibility is the ability to shift the focus of sampling as needed. For example, certain segments of the population (e.g., blacks, Hispanics, the uninsured, the elderly) can be oversampled by altering the NHIS subsampling process. Sample sizes for specific conditions also could be controlled by altering the size of the NHIS subsample that is screened or by oversampling provider visits for rare conditions in the provider surveys.[4] The flexibility tied to sampling needs is limited only by the difficulty that NCHS would have in making the design alterations and by the time it would take to implement them.

Current NCHS scheduling plans to field the existing provider surveys annually would not be altered if the panel's recommended design framework is adopted. Finally, the timing is right to make the kinds of changes required by this design, since in recent years design integration involving the NHIS has been given a priority within NCHS and since significant redesign work is currently under way for the two surveys in which the greatest impact of change would be felt (i.e., the NHIS and the NNHS).

IMPLEMENTATION STRATEGY

The panel recognizes that, despite its many potential benefits, adoption of the recommended design framework raises several important issues that would require careful examination and resolution prior to making final decisions on the details of the design.

Many of these issues are related to some of the screening and patient follow-up procedures. Perhaps the most important are: (1) to identify provider visits, (2) to obtain useful information to contact identified providers, (3) to obtain permission from the patients to peruse the provider records of those whom the NHIS respondents identify, and then (4) to successfully enroll the providers and the patients in the study.

Another important issue regarding the design of the proposed National Health Care Data System as recommended by the panel is the capacity to follow persons in receipt of care for a fixed length of time or until outcome, and in some instances beyond NHIS PSU boundaries. Follow-up might conceivably involve some combination of face-to-face and telephone inter-

---

[4]Other methods for sampling for rare conditions should also be investigated, including multiplicity or network sampling. A description of this and related methods and an introduction to related literature are included in Sudman and Kalton (1986); Kalton and Anderson (1986); Sudman et al. (1988); Nathan (1976); Sirken (1972).

viewing. Both modes have already been considered for use in the NHIS and the NMES. The telephone, for example, might be used only as a backup to the face-to-face follow-up if the person moves away from the area. Additional research into finding the most effective strategies for episode follow-up are necessary.

As discussed earlier, although the concept of episodes of illness is attractive and such data would prove to be a very valuable analytical database, especially for medical effectiveness research, experience with its application is limited and problematic. Developing the capability to generate data on episodes of various types of illness raises important and complex methodological issues associated with definition, classification, and measurement.

Finally the potential for difficulties with the process of linking large person-level data files from the persons' visited providers, their health care utilization, the process of care during an illness episode, and the final outcome should not be underestimated.

Recommendation 4-8: The panel recommends that NCHS establish a research agenda to determine the feasibility of its recommended course of action. If found feasible, the panel recommends that NCHS adopt the proposed design framework (with adjustments as warranted by the research) for a National Health Care Data System.

In conclusion, the panel recognizes two different, but not mutually exclusive, courses of action for establishing an integrated National Health Care Data System. The first course of action, put forth by NCHS, calls for limited geographic integration of the provider surveys with NHIS, extending the coverage of the provider surveys, and adding patient follow-up to the NHDS and the NAMCS. In effect, this plan envisions a collection of slightly modified provider surveys with follow-up components as the National Health Care Survey.

The panel believes this course falls short of meeting anticipated health information needs for the next century. It therefore proposes a different and more ambitious course of action, one that encompasses most of the features of the NCHS proposal, but also calls for a significant long-term expansion in the breadth and depth of information to be gathered through a comprehensive National Health Care Data System.

The section outlines below steps in a multiyear implementation strategy for the panel's proposed plan starting in 1992. The strategy is divided into four, at times overlapping, phases involving the initiation of the research agenda, developing and implementing the panel's design framework and recommendations for improvements in content and coverage of the information gathered, followed later by research into the feasibility of surveying episodes of illness and the associated patterns of care and outcomes.

Suggested Implementation Schedule

Phase I: 1992-1995

(1) NCHS begins work on the development and implementation of the panel's proposed design framework and the recommended improvements in the data content for the data system. Many aspects of the proposal have minimal impact on the designs of the underlying existing survey vehicles.

(2) NCHS initiates a research program to carefully consider the issues identified in the preceding sections of the report. NCHS should work in collaboration with the Agency for Health Care Policy and Research in researching the issues relating to the feasibility and efficacy of gathering data on episodes of illness.

(3) NCHS begins the process of convincing the Department of Health and Human Services, the Office of Management and Budget, and the Congress of the importance of this effort for federal health care policy and to ensure that this effort receives adequate funding and staff resources.

Phase II: 1995

NCHS begins implementation of the panel's recommendations with any modifications and adjustments as warranted by the research results to date.

Research agenda continues.

Phase III: 1994-1997

NCHS sets upon a one-year period to flesh out the design protocols for the panel's plan if found feasible in Phase I and with modifications as warranted by the results of the research.

NCHS begins developmental work for implementation of the panel's long-range proposal for surveying illness episodes.

Phase IV: 1997-2000

NCHS commences implementation of all components of the panel's proposed design framework for a comprehensive National Health Care Data System.

5

Coordination and Resource Considerations

The panel's recommendations in the previous chapters are intended to provide a considerably enhanced body of knowledge about the health and well-being of the U.S. population, the health care received, the costs associated with that care, and the relationships between the process and outcomes of care.

In the course of its study the panel has noted several issues not directly addressed in its charge, some broadly relating to activities of the National Center for Health Statistics (NCHS), and still others that go beyond to the structural issues of collaboration and coordination of data gathering and analysis within the Department of Health and Human Services (DHHS) as a whole. The panel strongly believes that these broader issues must be addressed in the context of this report because the successful implementation of an integrated and effective National Health Care Data System will to a large extent depend on their resolution.

ADVISORY STRUCTURE FOR THE NATIONAL HEALTH CARE DATA SYSTEM

NCHS, by legislative mandate, is the lead health statistics agency in the federal government. By no means, however, does it have the sole responsibility for all health statistics. A general purpose statistical agency such as NCHS cannot be all things to all people in the sense of fulfilling every potential user's information needs. The accepted role of the agency is the provision of a time series of comprehensive, timely, and reliable information on the health status of the population and the health care system. In pursuit of producing consistent baseline information over time, it is all too easy for statistical organizations to fall into at least two traps:

- To produce information conducive to making statistical generalizations but not sufficiently focused to provide detailed illumination of specific issues required to guide policy decisions and

- To produce information that is comparable over time but as a result has conceptual roots in issues or concerns of the past rather than those of the present.

To many people interviewed by the panel, the current Health Care Statistics program of NCHS has fallen into both of these traps to some extent—the current surveys generate primarily descriptive data about the supply side of the health care system, and provide only data of a secondary nature to anyone wishing to analyze health care policy or clinical or epidemiological issues. The information collected is often not sufficiently comprehensive. As noted previously, the current provider surveys focus on a unit of analysis—the event—which by itself is of declining relevance.

The panel argues that NCHS should continue to produce baseline information. NCHS also needs to redirect its resources and surveys within its statutory mandate to capture information relevant to current issues; provide a flexible capacity that will allow collection of more detailed or specific information on an ongoing basis. This issue is not unique to NCHS, as illustrated by W.G. Cochran in his discussion of the role of statistics in national health policy decisions in 1976:

> Any continuing general purpose survey may in time become outdated because it is unresponsive to changing needs as perceived by users when new problems arise. Criticism is sometimes directed toward the survey statisticians, who are accused of concentrating on what they believe to be their expertise: planning for the collection of samples and making estimates from them, without either interest or competence in judging the utility of what is being collected.

It has been 35 years since the passage of the National Health Survey Act (see Appendix D), yet the provisions of that law are as relevant today as they were in the 1950s. No far-reaching fundamental change in structure or the general organizational framework of the surveys has been made in response to changing health information needs since the early years, when the concept, operational definitions, and consequent organizational structure of the surveys were put in place. In fact, until the current efforts to develop a national health care survey, no new major survey had been developed within NCHS since the late 1970s. For various reasons, including resource constraints, the last major new surveys to be developed were the National Ambulatory Medical Care Survey and the National Medical Care Utilization and Expenditure Survey; the most recent successor of the latter, the National Medical Expenditure Survey, is not located in NCHS. Although much has changed since the 1970s in the health care system and in the sophistication of policy makers who demand and use these statistics, the surveys have not been able to keep pace with the changes and needs.

The panel believes that the concept and operations of major systems such as the recommended National Health Care Data System should undergo external review periodically by experts from outside the government. The panel of course recognizes the inherent practical and operational dilemma of a strong built-in bias for maintaining the status quo. Still, it is important to periodically reconsider, modify, and change as necessary in order to stay current and relevant.

A continuing, comprehensive, and integrated database is needed to analyze the policy issues surrounding the health care system, one that would serve the Congress, administrators, and other decision makers in the relevant federal agencies and the health care research community as well. The panel firmly believes that a redesigned National Health Care Data System as recommended in the previous chapter is an essential ingredient for significantly increasing the value of national health care data. Although the proposed design may be regarded by some as a substantial departure, with a gradual and small-scale approach more appropriate, in the panel's judgment exactly such an initiative is required to halt the drift toward becoming marginal and the inevitable further erosion of the NCHS health care statistics budget.

The panel therefore has recommended that NCHS begin *now* to implement its recommendations for a comprehensive integrated National Health Care Data System and to plan a steady incremental development throughout the remainder of the 1990s. Detailed specifications on the scope and content of an integrated National Health Care Data System that is responsive to the changing information needs will require concerted planning efforts, resources, and expert guidance and oversight.

Recommendation 5-1: The panel recommends that a continuing external oversight group of health care professionals be established to monitor and advise NCHS and the Department of Health and Human Services on the overall directions and scope and content of the National Health Care Data System, in the context of the agenda set forth by the panel in its proposed strategy for implementation.

The panel has provided a design framework for implementation by NCHS; it has also recommended that further research be undertaken on feasibility and methodological issues in order to reach informed decisions on implementing the details of the design. In the panel's opinion, NCHS would benefit from technical guidance provided by an external group of technical experts.

Recommendation 5-2: The panel recommends that an external technical committee of relevant experts be established during the planning and implementation phase to help plan and review the research needed to complete the proposed design; to identify the priorities for feasibility and research projects; and to monitor the progress made by NCHS in completing the research agenda and implementing the recommended design for a National Health Care Data System on schedule.

The technical committee could be part of the functions of the recommended oversight group for the National Health Care Data System or a separate working group functioning independently. The working group established under the auspices of the Section on Survey Research Methods of the American Statistical Association, which currently advises the Bureau of the Census on the Survey of Income and Program Participation, has been an effective vehicle for the Bureau; it could serve as a model for consideration by NCHS in carrying out the above recommendation.

IMPROVING DEPARTMENTAL COORDINATION

The panel has been impressed by the information-gathering capabilities that have been developed in other DHHS agencies, largely in response to their needs for data on which to base program decisions (see Appendix C). The panel is concerned, however, at the extent of fragmentation and what appears to be uncoordinated and at times overlapping development of health statistical activities in the department. It is not this panel's responsibility to say that these activities in the other agencies should or should not continue to exist, or to pass judgment on how all those activities relate or will relate to the proposed National Health Care Data System. It is the responsibility of the department, however, to ensure that statistical information needed for policy formulation is gathered, analyzed, and made available in a timely and cost-effective manner consistent with the mission and mandates of the department and its components without unnecessary duplicating and overlapping activities. Section 304 (c)(1) of the Public Health Service Act, requires the secretary to coordinate the health statistics activities undertaken and supported through the units of the Department of Health and Human Services. The panel concludes that the department needs to undertake, with expert consultations as needed, a major review of the vast array of its data collection activities related to health care with the objective of developing a comprehensive and coordinated plan for establishing an efficient and cost-effective structure and organization for health care statistics.

Considering the current fragmented state of the federal health statistics activities, unless such a review is conducted and the findings implemented, various agencies increasingly will fund special expensive one-time or periodic surveys to meet their specific needs, when in fact, well-designed and properly focused initiatives, conducted routinely, would meet many of those needs in a cost-effective manner. For example, better coordination and integration are needed than now exist between the kinds of data NCHS has traditionally collected, the administrative data that now are collected by Medicare and soon Medicaid, and the state-based data systems. The federal government needs current, relevant, and reliable data on the entire population in order to carry out its responsibilities conscientiously. It is especially important that ongoing dialogue and collaboration exist between the agencies, especially NCHS, the Agency for Health Care Policy and Research, the Health Care Financing Administration, and the Alcohol, Drug Abuse, and Mental Health Administration. Similar concerns have been expressed by others about the need for improved data on health care policy and the consequent need for coordinating and steering groups to determine priorities for development of data collection systems (see Citro and Hanushek, 1991, for a discussion on this subject).

Recommendation 5-3: The panel recommends that the Department of Health and Human Services establish an ad hoc external high-level committee, comprised of persons who have distinguished themselves in the field of health statistics, survey and sampling methods, and the provision of health services, to undertake a comprehensive review of the health statistics activities throughout the department and report its findings directly to the secretary.

Such a committee should have a budget and qualified staff support that is independent of all the agencies involved and well respected by all parties of interest. One possibility is to carry out this effort in collaboration with the National Committee on Vital and Health Statistics (NCVHS), which is the principal statutorily established advisory body to the secretary on health statistics matters. However, because of its size and the selection of its membership to be broadly concerned with health and vital statistics, it is not constituted to have the range of skills and technical expertise needed to undertake effectively the kind of task envisioned by the panel and other such activities. Furthermore, to undertake such a task, it would be essential to have additional ad hoc expert consultation when needed, a highly qualified independent staff, and an adequate operating budget. It is also essential, in carrying out such tasks, that the committee should report directly to the secretary as called for in the statute.

Even assuming that the department takes on this very comprehensive review, as stated earlier, major data systems still should be reviewed periodically. The panel believes that there should be some means of periodic review for the department to assess the capability and effectiveness of the statistical activities, looking at such matters as survey content, resources, and organization in the context of the nation's needs for health care information. One possible locus of such external accountability could be the NCVHS if strengthened along the lines indicated above.

In order for data collected by all agencies to be most useful, core data sets and concepts need to be comparable. NCHS should work in collaboration with the program agencies and the policy staff offices in the department in developing and encouraging the use of standard definitions and classifications and act in other ways to enhance the usefulness of the information and to reduce costs and unnecessary duplication of effort.

As indicated earlier, increased coordination and collaboration between the agencies in the collection, linkage, and analysis of health care data are essential. Medicare administrative data files increasingly have the capability of providing comprehensive information for the population age 65 and older. Special studies are being developed on the Medicare beneficiaries, Medicaid-eligible nursing homes, and other areas of interest and concern to the Health Care Financing Administration. Examples of such major initiatives are the Medicare Current Beneficiaries Survey, the Nursing Home Resident Assessment data set, and the Medicare health status registry. The panel recognizes, however, that data from administrative files are not necessarily substitutes for data from statistical surveys, and the two types of data are not always additive.

ENHANCING THE CENTER'S ANALYTIC CAPABILITY

Establishing and maintaining high-quality and relevant data systems for appropriate, timely dissemination requires a capable analytic staff of internal users. The panel finds that, although NCHS has maintained its emphasis on and capacity to ensure the validity and reliability of the data collected, there has been a loss of analytic capability, particularly within the survey divisions of NCHS for various reasons, but primarily as a result of budgetary constraints. At the very time that major health policy issues are being increasingly debated and policy and program managers and researchers in government and in the private sector are seeking better information for their purposes, the data appear to be becoming less pertinent to their needs. As a result, the users are turning to the stewards of administrative data such as the Health Care Financing Administration and the newly created Agency for Health Care Policy and Research for primary national data collection for which NCHS has the mandate and should have the capacity to provide.

In times of budget limitations, data analyses are often sacrificed to protect the basic data collection activities in a statistical agency. That is what appears to have happened in the survey divisions of NCHS over the past several lean budget years. The panel recognizes that NCHS does have a very strong but very lean separate Office of Analysis; however, the small staff of that office cannot, and should not, undertake all the analysis of the data from all the surveys. Strong analytic capability in the divisions that develop and conduct the surveys is important for keeping the content of the surveys relevant. The current impoverished analytical capability of these divisions not only affects the timely analysis and interpretation of data collected, but also leads to inability to anticipate important issues and to respond to them. The panel believes that, if not corrected, this will impair the ability of NCHS to implement the National Health Care Data System.

Recommendation 5-4: The panel recommends that the department ensure that sufficient resources for maintaining capability for analysis and dissemination of the data collected be included in the resources allocated for implementation of the National Health Care Data System.

RESOURCE REQUIREMENTS

Moving from event-based statistics to comprehensive person-based statistics, which the panel believes is absolutely essential for the provision of adequate health care data, cannot be accomplished without a substantial infusion of new resources. The panel feels that it would be remiss if it did not emphasize the importance of this additional funding and attempt to provide at least a crude estimate of what would be necessary to produce the recommended data on a continuing basis.

The lack of funding and staffing over the past several years at NCHS at a level adequate to even maintain the traditional survey infrastructure, let alone expand into new areas, methods and analysis, is extremely troubling to the panel. Inadequate funding has been translated into reduction in the frequency and sample sizes of surveys and, although harder to document directly, probably a decline in the quality and analytic utility of the surveys.

Health care data are of interest not only in terms of the broad functions of society, but also more importantly in terms of specific use and interest in the establishment and evaluation of federal policy in health care. The panel considers that the immediate implementation of its recommendations is justified in view of the increased importance of health care issues to Congress and the executive branch in the establishment and evaluation of federal health care policy, and to the states and the society as a whole as they cope with the significant changes in the organization and delivery of health care.

The National Health Care Data System as recommended by the panel must be funded adequately from the start if it is to be successfully designed, implemented, and operated. The panel recommends a considerably expanded data collection effort and a redesign strategy that will yield significantly more useful data than are currently available. An underfunded program cannot discharge its responsibilities effectively. In the final analysis, the commitment and institutional support of the secretary of the Department of Health and Human Services, the Office of Management and Budget, and the Congress are all essential to the successful implementation of a departmental comprehensive integrated health care statistics strategy.

The panel has proposed a strategy with a number of decision nodes in the future based on the results of the research agenda. Costs for implementing the coordinated data system proposed by the panel will depend on the decisions reached at the end of each stage. Implementation of the proposed design will take time and many of the specific details will emerge over the period. The panel therefore does not believe it is possible to provide precise estimates of funds needed to implement the proposed data system. However, on the basis of past and current expenditures for comparable national surveys conducted in the department, one can estimate the relative magnitude of funds that will be needed for data collection when the National Health Care Data System is operational.

Based on projected costs for fiscal 1992 and 1993, the annual cost of data collection for the provider surveys included in the current NCHS plan (excluding the patient follow-up component), is about $9-10 million.[1] This amount does not include any data processing, personnel, or overhead costs for these surveys. Comparable annual costs for the National Health Interview Survey are about $12 million. The National Medical Expenditure Survey contract costs for data collection were over $66 million for 1987-1989 (in 1987 dollars). This total includes $32 million for the household survey component, $11 million for the institutional population survey, $7.5 million for the medical provider survey, $9 million for the health insurance survey, $7 million for the survey of American Indians, and $.4 million for the medical record survey component. The panel estimates that, in 1991 dollars, these data collection contract costs would be in the range of $74-77 million, even with a modest rate of inflation of 3-4 percent per year.

The National Health Care Data System when fully implemented will include not only a largely expanded information base on providers and visits linked at the person level to the National Health Interview Survey, but also longitudinal components of the household and institutional populations linked to the National Health Interview Survey and the National Nursing

---

[1] The surveys included are the National Hospital Discharge Survey, the National Ambulatory Care Survey, the National Home Health and Hospice Care Survey, the National Health Provider Inventory (which will be conducted every three years; the last one was conducted in 1991), and the National Nursing Home and Board and Care Home Survey.

Home Survey, respectively, to obtain current information on patterns of health care utilization, costs, and expenditures—but in a more cost-efficient manner. On the basis of past and current experience with conducting similar surveys and taking into consideration potential cost savings resulting from its recommendations, the panel estimate that the annual data collection costs for the proposed integrated National Health Care Data System could be expected to be no less than $25-30 million (in 1991 dollars). This figure includes the $9-10 million currently estimated for the conduct of the provider surveys.

Recommendation 5-5: The panel recommends that adequate funds for operating the National Health Care Data System, estimated to be no less than $25-30 million per year, be included in the appropriated budget of the National Center for Health Statistics.

In conclusion, the panel believes that the blueprint for action that it recommends will contribute toward a significantly improved and efficient data collection system that will go far toward meeting the data needs for monitoring and evaluating the quality, access to, effectiveness and outcomes, and costs and expenditures for health care in the United States into the next century. The blueprint is worthy of full fiscal support, even in these difficult financial times, from the Congress and the executive branch.

APPENDIX A

The NCHS Plan for a National Health Care Survey

THE NATIONAL HEALTH CARE SURVEY

**Division of Health Care Statistics
National Center for Health Statistics
Centers for Disease Control
December 1990**

EXECUTIVE SUMMARY

During the past decade, notable changes in the organization, financing, and delivery of health care have occurred brought about, in part, by cost containment and medical effectiveness initiatives, aging of the population, and changes in the practice of medicine. Further changes are anticipated in the future. The impact of these changes includes a greater diversity in insurance and benefit programs; development and growth in new or alternative settings of health care; and changes in the medical care received by individuals and in the use of medical care technology.

These changes have outpaced the capabilities of existing data systems to provide relevant and timely data, a problem compounded by the periodic nature of many surveys. As a result, the National Center for Health Statistics (NCHS) has undertaken a major review of its existing surveys of health care providers. This review has evolved into plans for a restructuring of these surveys.

Under this plan, four NCHS surveys of health care providers, the National Ambulatory Medical Care Survey, the National Hospital Discharge Survey, the National Nursing Home Survey, and the National Master Facility Inventory, are being merged and expanded, over time, into an ongoing, integrated National Health Care Survey (NHCS). In part, this is being accomplished by reducing the sample sizes for health care providers covered in existing surveys and by stretching the sample over a number of years.

The primary objectives of the NHCS are: to provide national data for "alternative" sites of health care, such as hospital emergency and outpatient departments, ambulatory surgi-centers, home health agencies, and hospices; to increase the analytical uses of survey data through the use of an integrated cluster sample design; to develop the capability to conduct patient follow-up studies to examine issues related to the outcome and subsequent use of medical care; and to survey health care providers on an annual basis, thus eliminating gaps in data and fluctuations in resource requirements.

NCHS has requested that the Institute of Medicine and the Committee on National Statistics conduct a panel study to evaluate and make recommendations regarding the proposed plans for the National Health Care Survey.

TABLE OF CONTENTS

I. Background
   A. Dynamics of the Health Care Delivery System
   B. Impact on the Health Care Delivery System
   C. NCHS Data Systems
   D. Implications for Health Care Data

II. A National Health Care Survey
   A. Components
   B. Coverage
   C. Content
   D. Features
   E. Flexibility
   F. Integrated Survey Design
   G. Current Status and Schedule

I. BACKGROUND

A. Dynamics of the Health Care Delivery System

There have been profound changes in recent years that have reshaped many aspects of the health care delivery system in the United States. Further changes are expected to take place in the years to come. These changes affect not only the recipients of medical care, but the providers of care and medical insurance and benefit programs as well. Any overview of factors influencing the health care delivery system necessarily involves a degree of oversimplification; however, the following areas are among those frequently discussed:

Cost containment—Health care expenditures increased from $248 billion in 1980 to $500 billion in 1987, an increase of 102 percent, compared with a 66 percent increase in the Gross National Product. In response to these rapidly increasing health care expenditures, public and private purchasers of care have moved to institute reforms in the traditional third-party payment mechanisms, which were widely perceived as providing incentives for overutilization of health services. Major reforms by government have included the implementation of the Medicare Prospective Payment System; strengthening of Federally-mandated utilization review programs; State-initiated reforms in Medicaid programs; and physician payment reform. At the same time, businesses and insurance carriers, individually or through local coalitions, have moved to strengthen claims and utilization review; to institute greater cost sharing with beneficiaries; to offer expanded choices of coverage levels to employees, including capitation arrangements; and to use their market power to enter into preferred provider arrangements with hospitals and physician groups.

Medical effectiveness—Recent legislative and departmental health care initiatives, mirroring the feeling of many health care professionals, have focused on the effectiveness and outcomes of health care. Several activities indicating the importance of this emerging issue have occurred in the past year: Congress has enacted legislation to expand the Federal program of medical effectiveness research; and the Department of Health and Human Services, as part of its Medical Treatment Effectiveness Program, has awarded approximately $6 million in research grants to study patient outcomes and effectiveness of medical treatment. In September 1989, two "Effectiveness" conferences, including one sponsored by the Institute of Medicine, were held to review various aspects of this complex issue, such as the current research and health policy activities, the methods and data necessary for assessment, and the future direction of this effort.

Aging of the population—Rapid growth is occurring in the number and proportion of older persons in the population, as life expectancy at birth has risen to nearly 75 years; more importantly, persons reaching age 65 can expect, on average, to live another 17 years. Improvements in the morbidity status of this population have led to growing numbers that can live relatively independently, and a rise in the demand for health and social services that support independent living. At the same time, those persons that are institutionalized consume a large and growing share of health resources. This demand will expand in future years as the baby boomers age into the 65 years and older group.

Medicine and technology—Over the last several decades, investment in basic research, combined with a reimbursement system that encouraged the use of technology, has led to the rapid development and diffusion of new diagnostic and treatment modalities. In many cases, due to reimbursement incentives, intensity of treatment, and cost, the use of these procedures was limited to inpatient settings. In recent years, as many existing technologies have become more routine and new lower-intensity and less costly procedures have been developed, many procedures are now performed in outpatient and ambulatory settings. A variety of new facilities have emerged and grown to address this health care market.

B. Impact on the Health Care Delivery System

In the 1970's, the health care system was characterized by heavy reliance on inpatient care, fee-for-service physicians, cost- or charge-based reimbursement through third-party insurers, and the insulation of consumers of health care from financial risk. During the 1980's, as a result of some of the factors outlined above, there has been a growing trend toward greater diversification in organization, financing, and delivery of health care. Evidence of this diversity includes the proliferation of insurance and benefit alternatives for individuals; new forms of physician group practice; and growth in the number of alternative sites of care, such as surgical centers, walk-in ambulatory care facilities, and home health agencies.

Surgery is now provided on an outpatient basis for many procedures for which patients would have been admitted as inpatients previously. The substitution of alternative sites of medical care for high-cost inpatient hospital care is having a dramatic effect on the structure, organization, and finance of surgical care to the point that for some procedures the outpatient and ambulatory settings have become the preferred location for such care.

The emphasis placed on the reduction of regulation and promotion of market forces, as well as efforts to contain costs, has led to increased competition between providers and insurers of health care. At the Federal level, health planning programs have been de-emphasized, and other forms of regulation have been eased. At the same time, employers and insurers have facilitated increased competition by offering a greater range of choices, and consumers have responded with a growing acceptance of alternative forms of health care organization, as shown in the growth of enrollment in health maintenance organizations and other types of prepaid plans. Further, providers, in positions of both relative oversupply or underutilization, have sought to more aggressively market their services or enter into "preferred provider" arrangements to protect their market share.

One of the many emerging themes in the area of medical effectiveness research is the need for reliable and valid utilization data to measure and assess health care outcomes and medical technology. Discussion of these data needs and the methods for obtaining and analyzing these data is a frequent agenda item, for example, the use of administrative data and registries to assess medical effectiveness was explored at the IOM conference.

The aging of the population has led to concerns regarding the adequacy and cost of existing long-term care services, and a growing attention to long-term care insurance, as well as alternatives to institutionalization. The demand for long-term care services is exemplified by the dramatic rise in the number of nursing home beds in the 70s and 80s and an occupancy rate which has remained fairly constant over that time. And while home health care is often promoted as a cost-efficient alternative to institutionalization, there are concerns that more ready access to home health care will increase overall costs as new demand surfaces from individuals not currently receiving such assistance from organized providers.

Increasingly, health care institutions are becoming vertically integrated (wherein one firm or facility serves several provider functions, such as hospital, nursing home, and home health care) with greater likelihood of substitution between levels of service as individual patient needs or the availability of reimbursement dictate.

Finally, changes in the organization and financing of health care have resulted in significant changes in the practice of medicine and the development and use of technology. Since the implementation of the Medicare Prospective Payment System, lower inpatient lengths of stay have been observed, stimulating some debate over the extent of inappropriate early discharges; practitioners are placing more emphasis on the efficacy and cost effectiveness of technologies, where in the past any marginal benefit to the patient was sufficient justification for use of a procedure. Lower hospital occupancy rates again reflect the movement from inpatient to outpatient care. Greater emphasis is also being placed on early diagnosis and treatment of patients in capitation systems, while the increased employment of case management for Medicaid and privately insured groups has altered the traditional doctor-patient relationship in many settings.

C. NCHS Data Systems

Over its 30-year history the National Center for Health Statistics has developed and maintained, as changing data needs have dictated, a number of surveys of the supply, organization, and utilization of health care in the United States. These surveys have provided data for monitoring changes in the use of health care in these settings, for monitoring specific diseases, and for examining the impact of the introduction of new technologies. Examples include the data to examine the impact of the prospective payment system on the utilization of hospital care. The currently active surveys of health care providers are briefly described below.

The National Ambulatory Medical Care Survey (NAMCS), conducted annually from 1973-81, in 1985, and again on a continuous basis beginning in 1989, collects information about ambulatory medical care provided by office-based physicians. This survey provides statistics on the demographic characteristics of patients, reasons for visit, diagnoses, diagnostic procedures, services provided, drug therapy, and disposition.

The National Hospital Discharge Survey (NHDS), which has been conducted annually since 1965, is the principal source of information on inpatient utilization of hospitals. This survey obtains data on the characteristics of patients, their expected sources of payment, lengths of stay, diagnoses, surgical operations, and patterns of care by hospital bed size, ownership type and geographic region.

The National Nursing Home Survey (NNHS), conducted periodically since 1963 and most recently in 1985, provides information on nursing homes from two perspectives - that of the provider of services and that of the recipient. Data about the facilities include characteristics such as size, ownership, staffing patterns, Medicare/Medicaid certification, occupancy rate, days of care provided, and expenses. For residents, data are obtained on demographic characteristics, health status, services received and (for discharges) the outcome of care.

The National Master Facility Inventory (NMFI), conducted on a periodic basis since 1962, is an important source of national information on the number, type, and geographic distribution of inpatient health care facilities. In addition, the NMFI serves as a sampling frame from which facility samples such as the NNHS are selected.

These data systems rely on information from providers of health care, rather than from recipients, because 1) providers have the most accurate and detailed data on diagnosis and treatment, and 2) providers are an extremely cost-effective source for identifying events such as hospitalization, surgery, and long-term institutionalization, which are relatively "rare" events in the total population. For example, about 1 person in 10 receives hospital care each year and 1 elderly person in 20 uses nursing home care. Data from these surveys are obtained through a variety of mechanisms, including, for example, abstraction of medical records of institutions, completion of patient encounters by physicians, compilation of data from States and professional associations and purchase of data from private abstract services.

Other data systems provide important data on health care utilization, obtained from personal interviews with individuals. For example, the National Health Interview Survey provides data on physician and dental visits, as well as hospitalizations; and the National Medical Expenditure Survey (conducted by the National Center for Health Services Research) focuses on expenditures and financing of individuals for health care. These population-based surveys, while providing information on care received by individuals, are limited in their ability to provide accurate detail on diagnoses and treatments, or the characteristics of health care providers. On the other hand, these surveys do have the ability to obtain national estimates on expenditures for health care and insurance coverage, to provide information on persons who do not receive or have access to medical attention during a given period, and to provide socio-economic and health status information about respondents that is not readily available from health care providers.

D. Implications for Health Care Data

NCHS provider-based surveys have considerable strengths in measuring the care provided in traditional settings, including physicians' offices, acute care hospitals, and nursing homes. The NAMCS, NHDS and NNHS were designed to cover the health provider settings where the bulk of medical care was provided in the 60s and 70s. Despite the multitude of changes previously described, these sources of care remain as the key elements of the nation's health care data system. However, these data reflect only part of the medical care provided in the United States and, because of the kinds of changes previously discussed, there is concern that existing national health data sources are unable to fully address a number of areas of health policy interest, and are only partly capable of providing information needed to evaluate changes in the organization, financing, and delivery of health care. Current surveys are weak in two areas: (1) coverage of new and emerging sites of medical care, especially in those areas where new sites of care are substituting for the more traditional sources; and (2) measurement of the impact of change on the effectiveness, quality, and outcome of medical care.

Existing data systems are unable to measure the degree of shift from traditional to alternative settings, or to provide national estimates for types of care delivered in these new settings. Examples of these new or growing settings include hospital-based and freestanding ambulatory surgi-centers, ambulatory care provided in hospitals and clinics, and community-based long-term care settings. Furthermore, currently available estimates - such as rates for surgical procedures, physician visits and reasons for such visits, and receipt of long-term care - that are obtained from existing surveys may become less definitive as treatments and patients shift to other settings. A prime example of this shift is in the measurement of lens implants, which until recently were performed almost entirely as an inpatient service but are now performed with few exceptions on an outpatient basis. At the same time, data based on claims forms may become less useful as capitation systems gain larger market shares, since these systems require less detailed administrative records for reimbursement. In order to continue to provide basic estimates of the supply and use of health services and health care technology, surveys of health care providers will need to recognize the shift of medical practice to new settings.

Existing national data systems are limited in their ability to assess the impact of changes in the practice of medicine, such as the introduction of new technologies, and the resulting change in health outcomes that are brought about by modifications in financing and organization of such care. Important issues in this area include differences in health outcomes between different sites of surgery or other care in terms of subsequent institutionalization, mortality, or illness; differences in outcomes from alternative treatments or technologies employed for the same diagnosis; and the impact of declining inpatient lengths of stay for various diagnoses on subsequent readmission, other care, and on health outcomes.

The NCHS provider-based surveys were originally designed to operate continuously or with short periodicity cycles. Many of the problems of provider coverage described above have been compounded by the periodic schedule of data collection of some NCHS surveys of health care providers, for example, only the NHDS has been conducted on an annual basis during its entire history. Due to resource limitations, the scheduled interval between data collection periods in the NAMCS and NNHS were increased in 1981: the NAMCS from an annual to a triennial survey, the NNHS from triennial to sexennial. Further resource limitations led to the delay of these surveys from even the lengthened intervals. Although these programs are regarded as part of the NCHS base program, their periodic nature required justification of increased funding as each survey cycle approached. Despite the importance of these surveys to health researchers and policy makers, it has been increasingly difficult to obtain such funds. A more stable level of resources for surveys of health care utilization is required.

Finally, it is important to recognize the limitations of any analysis of current change in the health care system, and the danger of basing plans for future data collection solely on updating our current assessment of the structure of the delivery system. Change will continue to occur - both in reaction to the impact of previous changes and in response to forces that will emerge in the future. A critical concern as to future data collection is the flexibility to adapt to these changes as they occur.

II. A NATIONAL HEALTH CARE SURVEY

As a major initiative in the FY 1988 PHS Planning Process, NCHS examined the changes occurring in the health care delivery system, the impact of these changes, and the implications of these changes for the types of surveys of health care that are needed. The result is a plan for a major restructuring of its current surveys of health care utilization into a National Health Care Survey that is expected to provide a much more realistic picture of the medical care provided in the U.S. As the Center's four existing surveys of providers (the NAMCS, NHDS, NNHS, and NMFI) are fielded according to their projected schedule, they are being modified into components of the National Health Care Survey. Coverage of these surveys is being expanded to include alternative sites of care, and a greater continuity of resources is being achieved by moving periodic surveys to an annual basis. In part, this is being accomplished by reducing historical levels of sample size for health care providers covered in existing surveys and reducing or modifying the content of each provider component. The capability to conduct routine and specialized patient follow-up studies is being instituted through a patient follow-up component in order to address outcome and quality of care issues and greater analytic utility will be achieved through the use of an integrated cluster sampling approach. In the following sections the approach, features, and schedule for the National Health Care Survey are presented.

A. Components

The National Health Care Survey is designed to produce annual data on the use of health care and the outcomes of care for the major sectors of the health care delivery system. These data will describe the patient population, medical care provided, financing, and provider characteristics. The NHCS has five components based on the Center's current health care provider surveys:

The **Ambulatory Care Component** has as its base the National Ambulatory Medical Care Survey. This component is being expanded initially to include medical care provided in hospital emergency and outpatient departments and clinics. When fully implemented, this component will also cover ambulatory care provided in other settings such as neighborhood health clinics.

The **Hospital and Surgical Care Component** is based on the National Hospital Discharge Survey. This component is being enlarged to include hospital-based and freestanding ambulatory surgery centers.

The **Long-Term Care Component** is based on the National Nursing Home Survey and is being restructured and expanded to include home health agencies and hospices. The Long-Term Care Component will provide data from smaller annual surveys, rather than periodic surveys with larger samples.

The **Health Provider Inventory Component** is based on the National Master Facility Inventory. The NMFI which now provides the sampling frame for the NNHS and other facility based surveys is being expanded to include providers of acute ambulatory care and community-based long-term care. The NMFI has been renamed the National Health Provider Inventory (NHPI).

The **Patient Follow-up Component** is being developed to collect information from the patient or patient's family about the outcomes of patient care, including subsequent use of medical care and morbidity; hospital readmissions; and changes in health status. In this methodology periodic contacts (possibly by telephone) are made to follow the long-range outcomes of care and subsequent use of care to produce longitudinal data on quality of care, episodes of care and the dynamics of the use of health care and its financing. The application of this type of methodology in the 1985 NNHS is described in section G. Additionally, it is anticipated that these data could be linked with other data sources as the 1985 NNHS is being linked to the NCHS National Death Index to obtain information on mortality status and cause of death for former patients. The patient follow-up component could also focus on other dimensions: a financing mechanism, a diagnosis or procedure; a particular demographic group (e.g., aged, poor, minority); a particular disposition at discharge (e.g., live/dead, admission to long-term institutional care). The dimensions could change to address emerging issues and special topics.

B. Coverage

The National Health Care Survey is designed to cover the three major types of health care and health care providers:
Hospital Care:
- Inpatient
- Outpatient surgery
- Outpatient departments and clinics
- Emergency departments

Ambulatory Care:
- Physicians' offices
- Prepaid practice, including HMO's
- Freestanding surgi-centers

Long-Term Care
- Nursing and personal care homes
- Home health agencies
- Hospices

C. Content

Determination of the data content of the components of the National Health Care Survey is underway via discussions within the Department about basic data needs and research to develop specific data items. Traditionally, the basic core of data has been defined by an appropriate minimum data set - a common set of data items that meets the needs of a multiplicity of users. Several of these data sets have been designed by the National Committee on Vital and Health Statistics and it is possible that new data sets will need to be developed.

D. Features

Central to the development of a National Health Care Survey are several technical aspects or features which enhance its analytical capabilities and minimize costs. These features include:

> Employing an integrated cluster sample design where the health care providers are sampled at the second stage from a first stage sample of geographic areas, rather than selecting the providers at the first stage. Currently, the geographic areas being used in the NHCS are the Primary Sampling Units (actually a subsample of the PSUs) of the National Health Interview Survey. The advantages to this type of design include: the increased analytical utility as health care utilization is examined in relation to health status indicators; the reduced interviewing costs as sample providers are concentrated in specific geographic areas; the increased potential for record-linkage across settings which aids in tracking patients and in differentiating multiple episodes of the same condition; and the possibility of producing local area statistics, at least for some areas or communities.

> Conducting the components on a continuous annual basis to address seasonality of illness, to maintain a small group of well-trained staff, to reduce the budgeting and scheduling problems associated with periodic surveys, and to minimize recurrent start-up costs for survey components.

Using the same samples of providers over time, where possible, for better quality of data and reduced sample induction costs.

Using available data for developing sampling frames, e.g., for hospitals - the American Hospital Association; for physicians - the American Medical Association; and for certified home health agencies - the Health Care Financing Administration; and using the National Master Facility Inventory mechanism to complete or compile the sampling frames, e.g., surgi-centers, hospices and noncertified home health agencies.

Aggregating estimates across years to produce data on sub-populations, "rare" diagnoses and treatments, to produce greater geographic detail, and to compensate for smaller sample sizes.

As an example of other features which are being considered is the possibility of using the same sample of providers for several components of the NHCS, e.g., the same sample of hospitals might be used for surveys of inpatient, outpatient and emergency department care.

E. Flexibility

The National Health Care Survey is being designed for maximum flexibility, providing a basic framework which can be expanded in several dimensions as data needs change. This flexibility in an on-going national survey is important for providing data on changes in health care delivery such as new technologies, new procedures, and new approaches to organization or payment for care. Dimensions for expansion include:

Provider coverage—Coverage of health care providers can be expanded to include additional ambulatory and long-term care providers of interest, e.g., community health centers, walk-in acute care centers, adult day care centers, mental health facilities, or institutions for the mentally retarded. One the of general limitations for expansion is the availability and adequacy of a sampling frame.

Financing arrangements—In addition to source of payment, type of payment mechanism (fee for service, capitation, discounted fee, etc.) can be determined. As new payment mechanisms are implemented, the impact on the various sectors of the health care delivery system can be examined.

Special topics—The provider components and the patient follow-up component can be expanded to address special topics or emerging issues and can continue for several years if the issue warrants. Of current interest are the FY 1992 AIDS Initiatives which contain a concept proposal for the development and testing of a patient follow-up methodology.

Other applications of this longitudinal methodology include tracking the morbidity experience and subsequent use of services for patients hospitalized with stroke, or for patients in nursing homes with Alzheimer's Disease or hip fracture. And questions such as the following could be addressed: Do decreases in length of hospital stay for certain diagnoses result in greater use of long-term care or higher readmission rates to hospitals? What are the differences in morbidity and subsequent use of care when inpatient and outpatient surgery are compared for the same procedure?

F. Integrated Survey Design

As mentioned earlier, the components of the NHCS are being fielded in a subsample of the Primary Sampling Units selected for the National Health Interview Survey (NHIS). This linkage with the NHIS is consistent with the decision to base the NCHS Integrated Survey Design Program on the NHIS sample and to establish survey linkages to the other NCHS population surveys. The next cycle of NHIS redesign research is currently underway. Factors and design options now being explored include not only the issues related to the NCHS population surveys, but also the particular requirements of the NCHS provider and establishment surveys, e.g., the effect of conducting the NHCS in the NHIS PSU's and the analytical utility of such a design.

G. Current Status and Schedule

The current status and plans for the initial expansion of each NHCS component are described below and presented in Table 1. Also described are significant research and development activities previously completed.

Ambulatory Care

The 1989 NAMCS was redesigned based on the integrated cluster sample design (NHIS PSUs) and data collection began in March 1989. The 1989 and 1990 NAMCS samples include approximately 2,500 physicians in office-based practice. Data items will remain constant over the two-year period so that data can be aggregated to produce approximately the same level of detail as in 1985 when 5,000 physicians were sampled. Induction interview questions about health maintenance organizations and other prepaid practice arrangements have been incorporated into the 1989-90 NAMCS.

Based on the results of research conducted in two previous contracts which provided information on the availability of data items, appropriate data collection procedures, and construction of sampling frames, a contract is currently underway to develop the national sample design and conduct a field test to refine the data forms and collection procedures for the survey of hospital emergency and outpatient departments. This survey is scheduled to begin in mid-1991 and it is anticipated that the Bureau of the Census will be the data collection agent for the national effort.

Hospital and Surgical Care

The National Hospital Discharge Survey was redesigned based on the integrated cluster sample design and fielded in 1988. The redesigned NHDS sample contains 542 hospitals and emphasizes the purchase of discharge data from hospital abstract services as a method of data collection. Approximately 75 percent of the sampled discharges for the 1988 NHDS are collected via hospital abstract services. The design includes a nationally representative subsample of 128 hospitals which provide data on hard copy abstracts. This feature reduces the dependence on abstract services and provides narrative, as opposed to coded, diagnoses and procedures for special studies.

Research is currently underway via contract to develop a survey of ambulatory surgery centers. Among the technical and methodological issues being addressed in this research are the development of a data set and data collection procedures and the investigation of potential sampling frames. This survey would sample patients receiving surgical, diagnostic or therapeutic procedures in both hospital-based and freestanding ambulatory surgicenters. Implementation of this survey is currently scheduled for 1993.

Long-Term Care

Contract research is ongoing to develop a survey of clients of home health agencies and hospices. Data content and data collection procedures are being developed and a field test is currently underway. This work follows earlier work on the evaluation of the Long-Term Care Minimum Data Set which provided information on the establishment of sampling frames and on the content and availability of minimum data set items in agency records. Contingent upon the results of the current project, the home health agency/hospice client survey is scheduled to be pretested in late 1991 and fielded in 1992.

The schedule for the next National Nursing Home Survey has recently been accelerated so that the next NNHS will be fielded in 1992. It is anticipated that the Bureau of the Census will be the data collection agent.

Health Provider Inventory

Mailing lists of facilities for the 1991 National Health Provider Inventory are currently being prepared and in early 1991 the NHPI will be fielded. This mail survey will concentrate on compiling current and complete listings of home health care agencies, hospices, nursing homes, personal care homes and licensed board and care homes. The information collected will be used to construct sampling frames for the 1992 home health agency/ hospice client survey and the 1992 National Nursing Home Survey. Recommendations from a 1983-85 evaluation of the NMFI which addressed issues of definition, content, and data collection procedures for nursing homes and the experience from the centralized collection activities used in the 1986 Inventory of Long-Term Care Places conducted by NCHS are being incorporated in the 1991 NHPI.

Patient Follow-up

The 1985 NNHS included a survey of the current and discharged resident's "next-of-kin." This survey provided experience in obtaining release of information to identify the patient and in contacting the "next of kin" in order to collect longitudinal information not readily available in the medical record. This included information on the resident's health and functional status prior to admission, the reason for admission and a history of previous nursing home admissions. Two follow-up cycles have been conducted - one in 1987 (August-November) and the second in 1988 (July-October) - to determine the resident's current functional status, living arrangements, use of medical care and sources of payment since the last contact. A third follow-up cycle began in January 1990.

Future studies will rely on such work as the National Academy of Sciences evaluation of data needed for health policy analysis for an aging population which provides guidelines for the content of data items on quality and use of care.

TABLE 1 National Health Care Survey Implementation Schedule

Component	Year of data collection
	1988　1989　1990　1991　1992　1993　1994

Ambulatory Care
  Office-based physicians   X
  Hospital emergency and
    outpatient departments   X

Hospital and Surgical Care
  Hospital (inpatient)   X
  Surgical centers   X

Long-term Care
  Nursing homes   X
  Home health agencies and
    hospices   X

Health Provider Inventory
  Nursing homes   X
  Home health agencies   X
  Hospices   X
  Board and care homes   X
  Surgical centers   X

Patient Follow-up
  Nursing home residents X

APPENDIX B

Survey of Users of National Health Care Statistics

INTRODUCTION

Evaluation of plans for the National Health Care Survey requires detailed knowledge of the needs for the data that such a survey could produce. There is no systematic body of information about the users of NCHS data on health care or about the data needs of the users. In order to address its charge to evaluate plans for a National Health Care Survey, early in the study the panel decided to obtain the views of a wide group of users, policy makers, and other interested parties. Although the panel is comprised of experienced users of health care data and persons highly knowledgeable of the health care delivery system, it wanted to learn from users about the kind of health care data they use; how they use the data; their experience in using data from the current NCHS provider surveys (the National Hospital Discharge Survey, the National Ambulatory Medical Care Survey, the National Nursing Home Survey, and the National Master Facility Inventory); the problems they have encountered in doing so; their assessment of their quality, cost, and accessibility; their current needs for data on health care and their anticipated future needs; and their comments on the NCHS plans for the integrated National Health Care Survey.

As a first step in this direction, the panel decided to conduct an informal survey of users. The information obtained from users had significant influence on the panel in formulating its recommendations. The proposed

National Health Care Survey, however, cannot meet all the needs for data of all persons. Choices had to be made in terms of costs and benefits associated with policy making in the public and private sectors, as well as the burden on the public. The panel takes full responsibility for the ways in which the users' views have been considered and incorporated in the recommendations.

METHOD OF DATA COLLECTION

The panel had neither the time nor the resources to conduct a large-scale structured user survey designed to meet the standards of survey research. The panel therefore obtained the views of users through (1) presentations at panel meetings by key users of health care data and policy officials, mostly from the Department of Health and Human Services and some from the private sector and (2) through focused group interviews of selected federal health officials, legislative staff, researchers, and state vital and health statisticians.

Approximately 75 users and some nonusers representing the executive and legislative branches of the federal government, health statisticians and vital registrars from several states, and individual researchers in the private sector participated in the survey. The panel recognizes the limited nature of its efforts to obtain the views of users. For instance, the group interviewed is not necessarily representative of all current and potential users of NCHS health care data. Moreover, the expressed needs for data often reflect the mission of the agency interviewed.

The interviews were conducted in group sessions with the aid of an open-ended interview guide rather than a structured questionnaire; it appears at the end of this appendix. The guide was adapted to the needs and functions of the specific group interviewed and to the responses received during the specific interview. For several of the interviews, once the purpose of the interview was explained, it rapidly became an open-ended discussion. Nevertheless, attempts were made to ensure that all of the areas in the interview guide were covered even in this type of discussion. The areas in which questions were asked included the following:

Uses of data from the NCHS
Problems with uses of the data
Current data needs
Health care and health status issues of most concern for the next few years
Knowledge of NCHS plans for an integrated National Health Care Survey
Views on various features of the survey, such as:
    Coverage of the survey
    Content of the survey

Longitudinal data
Geographic detail
Data on subpopulations
Other.

Initial contact was made with the group to be interviewed by telephone, followed by a confirmation letter and information about the panel study and the nature of the inquiry. For the few persons who could not attend the group sessions, information was obtained by telephone interview.

The decision was made to concentrate mostly on federal agencies in the Washington, D.C., area. The following is a list of agencies that were represented in interviews:

Agency for Health Care Policy and Research, PHS
Alcohol, Drug Abuse, and Mental Health Administration, PHS
Office of the Assistant Secretary for Planning and Evaluation, DHHS
Health Resources and Services Administration, PHS
Social Security Administration, DHHS
Health Care Financing Administration, DHHS
National Institute for Occupational Safety and Health, CDC, PHS
National Institute of Diabetes and Digestive and Kidney Diseases, NIH, PHS
National Institute on Aging, NIH, PHS
Staff, House Subcommittee on Health and Environment
State health agencies in Connecticut, New York, Pennsylvania, North Carolina, South Carolina, Iowa, Michigan, Utah, Wisconsin, Maine

In addition, several individual data users from the private sector were interviewed.

FINDINGS

The survey of users of health care data was not a scientific sample and the results cannot be expressed statistically. Therefore, the findings are summarized in narrative form on the basis of responses to questions as well as unsolicited comments from the respondents.

Uses of Existing NCHS Provider Surveys

Most of the respondents were familiar with the four provider surveys, but not equally familiar with all four. Almost all of the groups interviewed had used data from at least one of the surveys. A majority of those interviewed responded that they were more familiar with the National Health Interview Survey (NHIS) and the National Nursing Home Survey (NNHS) than with the National Hospital Discharge Survey (NHDS) and had used, or are currently using, data from these surveys more than the other provider surveys.

The respondents were asked in what format or media do they usually obtain the data from NCHS. Published data and special tabulations appeared to be the usual format, followed by public use tapes, reflecting the heavy users of the data.

During the course of the interviews, the respondents were asked to describe the uses of the data and their experiences in using the data from these surveys. In responding, they tended to focus primarily on the problems they encountered in using the survey data, often for purposes for which the data were not specifically intended.

Many of the uses of the data were ad hoc applications to obtain answers to specific questions. The following are provided as illustrative examples of uses of the NCHS health care data and are by no means intended to be exhaustive.

- Analysis of hospital utilization rates by diagnosis and the distribution of procedures performed.
- Descriptive analyses of data on specific diseases—for example, hospitalization for diabetes using NHDS, the extent of ambulatory care for diabetes using NAMCS, and some aspects of cost of care for diabetes using the NNHS.
- Use of the NHDS for a study of hip fractures.

Problems Encountered With the Data

The respondents mentioned a number of problems that they encountered with the data from the current provider surveys. In general, these problems reflected the needs of the agencies for data that were not being met at the present time. To some extent, therefore, the list of problems reads like a list of data needs. The following list is illustrative of the problems surfaced for each of the provider surveys.

National Hospital Discharge Survey

- The survey is not person-based. It samples discharges and therefore does not measure what happens to individuals. There is no information on multiple admissions, the patient's contact with other providers, and the episode of illness.
- There is no information on disposition following discharge from the hospital.

- There is no information on payers or on cost of care.
- Information on race/ethnicity is not very useful because of a high proportion of "unknowns."
- There is no information on occupation of the person discharged.
- There is no hospital identification that would permit linkage to other data sets.
- The sample size is inadequate to produce estimates for small geographical levels, subgroups of the population, and relatively rare events.
- There is insufficient detail in the item content and lack of depth in the topics covered.

National Ambulatory Medical Care Survey

- Visits, not persons, are sampled, so there is no information on other contacts with this or other providers.
- There is no information on outcomes of care.
- There are no data on cost of care—only on source of payment.
- More diagnostic information is needed—five diagnoses rather than three.
- There is no information on occupation.
- Diagnostic data are outdated.
- There are no data on practice of providers and on their characteristics.
- There is no information on the other providers who assisted the physician.
- The survey does not include data on physician contacts with patients in the hospital.
- The sample size is too small.
- The survey is conducted at too infrequent intervals.

National Nursing Home Survey

- The survey does not sample persons.
- There are no longitudinal data on the person's condition or events and circumstances before and after the specific nursing home stay.

- The payer information is inadequate.
- The sample size is too small for many purposes.
- Data on subpopulations are inadequate.
- The rates of refusals and nonresponse are too high.
- The 8-year gap between surveys is too long.

National Master Facility Inventory

The National Master Facility Inventory serves as the sampling frame for the provider surveys. The overriding comment on the part of the users was that the coverage of the inventory was incomplete. The list of providers that the users proposed for inclusion are discussed below in the section on coverage of the proposed survey.

Looking Ahead to the National Health Care Survey

Looking ahead to the next few years, respondents were asked (1) what aspects of health care and related health status issues they will be most concerned with and (2) to comment on the features of the proposed integrated National Health Care Survey that would best meet their needs for data.

Key issues of concern in the years ahead identified by respondents are summarized below:

- Uninsured and underserved people.
- The aging population, long-term care for the elderly and nonelderly, care for the aged and cost of care to the aged, incidence and prevalence of chronic illness, disability, access to home health care.
- The impact of changes in financing policies on patients and on quality of services, access to care, and outcomes of care.
- Costs of prescription drugs.
- Income and expenditure data for health care, including long-term care.
- The extent of shifts from inpatient hospital care to ambulatory care. Costs and outcomes of care in inpatient and ambulatory settings.
- Access to care for HIV-infected persons, including adolescents, children, and those in rural areas.
- Effects on health habits and lifestyles of prevention programs.

The respondents were asked what features would make the proposed integrated National Health Care Survey best meet their needs for data. The sections that follow summarize under several topic headings the comments of the respondents on the features of the proposed survey that would best meet their needs for data.

Content. Almost all the groups interviewed expressed a need for data on the cost of health care. The subject was raised in the context of information on health insurance, out-of-pocket expenditures, managed care, types of providers, etc. Although some of these questions can be answered by data from the large national surveys such as the National Medical Expenditure Survey, these surveys are conducted too infrequently and the results of these surveys become outdated very rapidly because of changing costs, changes in financing of health care, changes in settings for specific kinds of care, etc.

Some of the groups interviewed were interested in the number and characteristics of the medically uninsured, the extent to which they move in and out of insurance coverage, what medical care, if any, they receive, and in what settings.

Person-based versus provider-based data. As indicated earlier, almost all of the users interviewed indicated the need for data on the health care received by individuals. This included health care received from a range of providers for specific conditions, costs of such care, etc.

Coverage. The respondents to the survey of users suggested 37 different types of providers not now being surveyed by NCHS that should be considered for inclusion in the National Health Care Survey:

    Adult day care centers
    Alcohol and drug abuse centers
    Board and care homes
    Chiropractors
    Chronic disease hospitals
    Emergency clinics
    Endoscopy units
    Foster care
    Group and residential care facilities
    HMOs
    Home care facilities
    Homes for the aged
    Hospices
    Hospital outpatient services
    Managed care facilities

Maternal and child health clinics
Mental hospitals
Mentally retarded facilities
Neighborhood health centers
Orphanages
Podiatrists
PPOs
Private insurance claims data
Psychiatric social workers
Psychiatric nurses
Psychologists
Psychosocial rehabilitation centers
Public health clinics
Radiology units
Rehabilitation medicine units
Retirement facilities
Rural health centers
Shelters
Surgical centers
Veterans Administration facilities
Visiting nurses
Walk-in clinics

Some of the providers on the list are already under consideration by the NCHS for inclusion and others are already included in surveys being conducted by other agencies.

Frequency. Very few of the respondents to the survey of users mentioned the frequency of data collection for the proposed survey. The comment most often heard in this area was that 8 years was much too long a gap between National Nursing Home Surveys.

Unit of analysis. The basic issue here is whether data collected should be based on a sample of events, such as doctor visits or hospital discharges, on characteristics of providers, or on persons and the medical care they receive. The primary interest of most of the users surveyed was in data on individuals in order to be able to answer questions about episodes of illness, costs of care over specific periods of time, the use of multiple providers, transition from one type of facility to another, access to health care, etc.

Several users were interested in data on providers in order to get basic information on the supply of health resources, including characteristics of providers, staffing patterns of providers, number of new nursing home beds, etc. Most also wanted some information on medical care events in addition to the data on individuals in order to measure the volume of care. They wanted more detailed information than presently available on the cost of service, sources of payment, specifics of services provided, etc.

Geographic detail. The estimates made from the current NCHS provider surveys are for the national level and for four broad regions of the United States. The respondents were asked at what geographic level they need data. Only a few indicated that they were interested only in national level data, and several felt that the four regions were too broad. Many wanted data at the state level, and several have need for data at the county or community level and for rural areas.

Subpopulations. Most of the respondents were interested in data for specific subpopulations: blacks, Hispanics, Asians (and specific subgroups of Hispanics and Asians), American Indians, disabled children, agricultural populations, specific industrial groups, older workers, disabled workers, children in general, groups defined by socioeconomic level, elderly, and nonelderly in institutions.

Longitudinal data. In most of the user interviews the question of their need for longitudinal data was raised. The term *longitudinal* was used in at least two ways: (1) Following a cohort of the general population to assess their use of the health care system over a period of time or (2) Following a cohort of persons seen by a particular type of provider to assess outcome or to determine what additional care they received from the entire range of providers over a period of time. Each of these approaches implies obtaining information from respondents about the health care they received over a period of time and then obtaining more specific information from their providers.

Several of the respondents expressed the need for longitudinal data on health care to serve a variety of purposes. The most common of these was to be able to assess episodes of illness, which would involve following individuals through the health care system as they had contacts with providers for specific conditions. Respondents in three group sessions indicated the need for data on outcomes of health care. However, they were not specific about what measures they would use and for what purpose, suggesting the need for specification of meaningful measures of outcome and the design of the longitudinal aspects of the health care survey to obtain such measures. One of the examples given was to be able to follow a cohort of persons discharged from hospitals to assess the extent of subsequent hospitalization, contacts with other providers, or death. Several of the respondents recognized two critical problems in obtaining longitudinal data on health care: (1) the need for identifiers on the individuals to be followed and their informed consent to allow their information to be linked with other data sets and (2) the cost of conducting follow-up surveys. Some concern also was expressed about the possible risk of jeopardizing other parts of the survey because of the cost of carrying out longitudinal studies of health care.

Linkage. On the subject of linkage with other data sets, most of the respondents wanted to see linkages not just with other NCHS databases, but with social security records, HCFA databases, and several databases in the private sector. It was recognized that, in order to link the databases, identifiers will be needed.

SURVEY OF USERS

Panel on the National Health Care Survey

Guide for Interviewing Users of Health Care Statistics

THE FOLLOWING SHOULD BE USED ONLY AS AN OPEN-ENDED GUIDE, TO BE ADAPTED TO THE NEEDS AND INTERESTS OF THE SPECIFIC GROUPS AND TO THE RESPONSES RECEIVED.

[The meeting will begin with an introduction and a five minute background of the study, the objectives of the session and the surveys covered in the questions.]

Current Data Needs

1) What aspects of health care and related health status issues are you currently most concerned with?

2) What kinds of programmatic action, policy decisions or research products result or could result from your work in this area?

3) What types of statistical information do you require to carry out analyses and or make decisions in this area?

Use of Data from NCHS

4) Have you used, or are you currently using, any data from NCHS on these subjects?

    User _____   Nonuser _____

                        IF NONUSER GO TO QUESTION 14

5) Are you a user of any of the following NCHS surveys of health care?

- National Master Facility Inventory or Inventory of Long-Term Care Places
- National Hospital Discharge Survey
- National Ambulatory Medical Care Survey
- National Nursing Home Survey

    yes _____   No _____

IF YES, ASK WHICH SURVEYS. IF NO, GO TO QUESTION 14

Questions for Users

6) In what format or media do you usually obtain these data — publications, special tabulations, public use tapes, etc. ?

   IF PUBLIC USE TAPES ARE USED ASK:

   - How many tapes have you used in the last 2 years?_____
   - Are you on the mailing list for NCHS publications?

   yes _____   No _____

   FOR EACH OF THE HEALTH CARE SURVEYS THAT YOU SAID YOU USE:

7) What uses have you made, or do you make, of data from this survey?

8) What end products derive from your use? (testimony, policy papers, review of legislative proposals, budget estimates, reports, research papers, etc.) Obtain some citations, if possible?

9) What do you consider to be the strong points of these surveys?

Problem Areas

10) What do you consider to be the weak points of these surveys?

    IF NONE, GO TO QUESTION 14

11) What kinds of problems have you encountered in attempting to use data from these surveys?

    WHICH OF THESE SURVEYS?

12) Have you had projects for which these surveys should be uniquely suited but cannot be used because of problems of design or lack of relevant data elements or sample size or other problems?

    IF YES, ASK TO ELABORATE

    Do you have any suggestions for solving these problems?

13) Do you use other sources of data in these subject areas?

    IF YES, WHAT ARE THEY?

Looking Forward

14) Looking ahead to the next few years, what aspects of health care and related health status issues do you think that you will be most concerned about?

15) For the past few years NCHS has been developing an integrated national health care survey including a follow-up component. Have you been aware of NCHS plans for an integrated National Health Care Survey ?

 yes _____ no _____

IF NO, BRIEFLY DESCRIBE

The new survey might include information covering a number of topic areas:

- Health care facilities
- Health care services provided
- Health manpower
- Recipients of health care
- Outcomes of health care
- The context within which the care is provided

16) Do you think data on any of these topics will be of particular interest to you—which ones and for what purposes—should any other topics be considered?

17) From your perspective what features would make the proposed integrated National Health Care Survey best meet your needs for data?

   a. Let's discuss *coverage* issues first. Do you have any thoughts on which facilities and places should be covered in this new National Health Care Survey ?

   b. Turning to the *content* of the survey, we are especially interested in those areas that are emerging or are of increased importance. What content areas should be covered in the new survey?

   c. How *frequently* do you need the data you mentioned earlier?

   d. Some data uses require *longitudinal* estimates, tracking changes over time for the same respondents. To what extent are longitudinal data needed in the area of health care statistics?

PROBE FOR SPECIFIC EXAMPLES

Some data needs suggest different approaches to survey design. One in particular that we seek your views on is *unit of analysis.* In the area of health care surveys, the unit of analysis may be *facility* (hospital, nursing home, doctor's office), *event* (admission, discharge, visit, particular services), or *person* (patient, client):

e. From your viewpoint, how important is it to obtain data on the facility? event? individual? For what kinds of analyses would data on each of these be important?

Another feature of interest may be *geographic* detail.

f. Are national data sufficient for your purposes, or do you need data for geographic subdivisions? If the latter, in what geographic detail?

IF RESPONSE IS "SMALL-AREA" OR "LOCAL," PROBE FOR DEFINITION

g. Do you need information on any specific *subpopulations?*

WHICH GROUPS?

h. Are there any *other* features you feel should be addressed in the review of the National Health Care Survey?

18) Are there other sets of data to which you would wish to link data from the National Health Care Survey?

IF YES, WHAT ARE THEY?

Can you give examples of how these data would be used - that is, what kinds of programmatic actions, policy decisions or research products might result from an analysis of the data?

What identifiers would be needed for the linkage —Social Security number, Medicare number, Medicaid number, or something else?

Do you see any problems in obtaining them?

19) In what format should data be made available in the future?— published reports, data tapes, special tabulations, or any other media?

WRAP UP

APPENDIX C

Federal Health Data Sources

The United States possesses one of the world's leading statistical systems, its current status having evolved over the course of the nation's history. As the role of the federal government has increased over the years, so has the demand for more and better statistics at the national and subnational levels. The federal statistical system in the United States is decentralized, with authority and responsibility for statistical activities spread among several agencies of the government.

There exists an abundance of statistical information related to the health status and the health care industry of this nation. A number of federal and state agencies gather and use health-related data. The private sector is also a major collector and user of such data. Yet, as shown in the body of the report, the current national data systems do not provide the information needed to assess the effect of changes in the financing, organization, and delivery of health care or the impact of socioeconomic trends on the quality, cost, and outcomes of care.

An understanding of the strengths and weaknesses of the current status of federal statistics and the prospects for continued development and progress in future years requires knowledge of the genesis of these systems and an understanding of the social, economic, public health and political factors that have led to a gradually increasing involvement of both the executive and legislative branches of the federal government in the collection and maintenance of health statistics.

EVOLUTION OF FEDERAL HEALTH STATISTICS

For many years after the formation of the federal union, responsibility for the collection of statistics in the health field was located primarily at the level of the state and local governments. Federal involvement was limited to a large extent to meeting the information needs for the most pressing health and related problems affecting the country and to the collection of vital records from the states.

Notification of diseases in this country began in the colonial times at the local level, particularly in port cities. However, the collection of the data was limited to times when epidemics of pestilential diseases threatened or were in progress. Statewide notification was first instituted in 1883, when Michigan passed a law requiring reporting of certain diseases (Bureau of the Census, 1960).

In response to the need for nationwide information on epidemic diseases, Congress passed a law in 1878 authorizing the collection of morbidity reports for use in connection with quarantine measures against pestilential diseases such as cholera, smallpox, plague, and yellow fever. This law was the start of the responsibilities of the Public Health Service (PHS) in the collection of data on communicable diseases and the surveillance of the incidence and distribution of diseases. A year later, a specific appropriation was made for such collection.

In 1893, Congress passed another law that provided for the collection of information each week from state and municipal authorities throughout the United States.

By the 1950s national health data sources were primarily comprised of the reporting by state and territorial authorities of morbidity statistics for communicable diseases and their surveillance and the death registration system. Completeness of reporting continued to vary greatly, and many illnesses were not reported to the authorities. Various health programs produced statistics specific to their programs, but they were neither national in scope nor comparable for different states. Current data that were representative of the general health status of the U.S. population were not available regularly.

A national health survey was conducted by the Works Project Administration in 1935-1936 as part of a comprehensive National Health Inventory, covering 700,000 urban families in the depressed economic conditions of the time. The survey had two purposes—to promote knowledge of the population's health status and to create jobs for the unemployed.

Twenty years later, statisticians inside and outside the government were still relying primarily on the 1935-1936 National Health Survey and a series of supplemental studies carried out in the 1940s and early 1950s as the basis for estimating the current level of illness and disability in the United

States.[1] Those data had become outdated. During the interim much had happened to change the country, the people, and their health status. The Great Depression was over; the country had gone through a major war and had recovered; the population of the United States was more urbanized; medical care had advanced and the people's health had improved.

During that period major advances had been made in statistical survey theory and methodology. The late 1940s and the early 1950s saw a series of local surveys conducted by various state and private organizations to study morbidity, disability, and handicapping conditions. Many of these studies broke new ground but none was national in scope. The Bureau of the Census and the PHS had provided advice to those carrying out these local surveys.

It was clear by the early 1950s that the federal government's role in health statistics could best be carried out by providing leadership in development of a national health data resource based on the probability sampling of households.

The National Health Survey Act

In 1953 the National Committee on Vital and Health Statistics (NCVHS)[2] recommended that a national health survey be established on a permanent basis. (NCHS, Ser.4, No.5, 1966) In 1956 Congress enacted PL 84-652, the National Health Survey Act (reproduced in Appendix D). The act authorized a three-part program: a continuing survey using probability sampling methods, special studies, and methodological studies. It authorized the surgeon general to make available technical advice and assistance on the application of statistical methods in health and medicine.

The content of the program of the National Health Survey was influenced by the varied nature of the data needed and the requirement in the act that corresponding information be obtained for both the well and the ill population. The National Health Survey was conceived as a program of surveys, with its objectives and approaches being flexible to adapt to changing needs for data and advances in statistical method. The activities of the National Health Survey as it is currently comprised are divided into three

---

[1]These studies were supplements to the Census Bureau's Current Population Survey, requested by the Social Security Administration and the Public Health Service. The supplement in 1943 (repeated in 1949 and 1950) dealt with the prevalence of disability, and another in 1951 dealt with the prevalence of arthritis. These were the first applications of national probability sampling of the population to the measurement of health.

[2]The U.S. National Committee on Vital and Health Statistics was established in 1949 by the surgeon general of the U.S. Public Health Service to put into effect a recommendation of the First World Health Assembly. On July 23, 1974, this committee was legislatively established under Section 306(k) of the Public Health Service Act (PL 93-353).

major parts, with data collected from three major types of sources. These are (1) the Health Interview Survey, (2) the Health Examination Survey, and (3) the Health Records Surveys.

A year after the passage of the National Health Survey Act, the Household Health Interview Survey (later renamed the National Health Interview Survey) began with the objective of producing general data on the nation's health. For several years this Household Health Interview Survey was the only major activity of the National Health Survey while the special studies also authorized by the law were being developed. In 1959, a second major component of the National Health Survey, the Health Examination Survey, was started, aimed at gathering health data by means of a physical examination of a sample of the population, and reached full-scale data collection by spring 1961. Special studies also authorized by the law were being developed. By 1961 several of the survey activities had begun that later made up the Health Records Survey program.

CURRENT DATA SOURCES[3]

The federal health statistics system, like the federal statistics system as a whole, is decentralized across the federal government. The majority of health statistical activities are undertaken by the Department of Health and Human Services, although the Department of Defense, the Veterans Administration, the Environmental Protection Agency, the Bureau of Labor Statistics, and other agencies collect and use health statistics in carrying out their respective functions.

Within the Department of Health and Human Services, the organization and decision-making structure for health statistical activities is further decentralized among the various organizational components of the department that have distinct responsibilities for gathering data directly related to their program responsibilities.

The section below briefly describes the data systems that these agencies operate that either contribute, or could contribute, to the understanding of the dynamics of our health delivery system and its impact on the health status of the American people. No attempt is made to provide an exhaustive listing or summary of all the health statistical activities carried out by federal agencies and programs. Only selected statistical activities of the National Center for Health Statistics (NCHS) and the department relevant to this present study are described.

---

[3]The information in this section is based on, and excerpted from, publications and other documents of the agencies of the federal government. These sources are provided at the end of the report.

National Center for Health Statistics

NCHS is the focal federal agency for the production, analysis, and dissemination of general-purpose health statistics. It is recognized as one of the principal statistical agencies of the federal government. The center was established in 1960 when the National Office of Vital Statistics and the National Health Survey Program in the Division of Public Health Methods were placed in one agency within the U.S. Public Health Service. Since its creation, the center has been moved to various locations within the organizational structure of the Public Health Service. Most recently, in 1987, it was placed as one of the Centers in the Centers for Disease Control (CDC).

Section 306 of the Public Health Service Act establishes the center in the Department of Health and Human Services and specifies that it shall collect statistics on:

- The extent and nature of illness and disability of the population of the United States (or of any groupings of the people included in the population), including life expectancy, the incidence of various acute and chronic illnesses, and infant and maternal morbidity and mortality;

- The impact of illness and disability of the population on the economy of the United States and on other aspects of the well-being of its population (or such groupings);

- Environmental, social, and other health hazards;

- Determinants of health;

- Health resources, including physicians, dentists, nurses, and other health professionals by specialty and type of practice, and the supply of services by hospitals, extended care facilities, home health agencies;

- Utilization of health care, including (1) ambulatory health services by specialties and types of practice of the health professionals providing such services and (2) services of hospitals, extended care facilities, home health agencies, and other institutions;

- Health care costs and financing, including the trends in health care prices and cost, the sources of payments for health care services, and federal, state, and local governmental expenditures for health care services; and

- Family formation, growth, and dissolution.

National Health Interview Survey

The National Health Interview Survey (NHIS) is the principal source of information on the general health status of the civilian, noninstitutionalized population of the United States. The NHIS is a cross-sectional household interview sample survey conducted annually since 1957. Interviews are conducted each week throughout the year. The survey follows a multistage probability sampling of households. It is designed in such a way that the sample scheduled for each week is representative of the target population and the weekly samples are additive over time.

The NHIS redesign in 1985 included a reduction of the primary sampling units (PSUs) from 376 to 198 for sampling efficiency and an oversampling of the black population. Data are collected from approximately 50,000 households including about 130,000 persons in a calendar year.

The survey provides national estimates on the incidence of acute illness and accidental injuries, the prevalence of chronic conditions and impairments, the extent of disability, the use of medical services, and other health-related topics by demographic and socioeconomic characteristics.

The questions in the core part of the questionnaire are asked each year. They solicit information to measure illness and injuries, days of disability including bed-days, work-loss days, school-loss days, and other days lost due to acute or chronic conditions. Included in the core are questions on limitation of activity caused by chronic conditions or impairments, hospitalizations, doctor contacts, perceived health status, as well as the social, economic, and demographic characteristics of the interviewed person. Questions on dental visits were also part of the core from 1975 through 1981.

The core questionnaire includes six lists of chronic conditions. Each condition list concentrates on a group of chronic conditions involving a specific system of the body, such as digestive, skin and musculoskeletal, circulatory, and respiratory. Prior to 1978, questions on only one condition list were asked each year. Beginning in 1978, each of six representative subsamples has been asked questions based on one of the six lists of chronic conditions. In this manner national estimates on each of the six body systems are obtained during the same interview year.

Questions on current health topics are included in supplements to the core questionnaire and change from year to year. They have been included in the NHIS since 1959, permitting the survey to collect information on a wide variety of health topics and to be responsive to the country's changing information needs. Because a supplement is added to the ongoing NHIS, which is an established vehicle resulting in statistically reliable data for the U.S. population, it is an efficient way to measure on a large scale and in a timely manner a topic of current concern. Some supplements, such as health insurance and out-of-pocket health expenditures, are repeated periodically to allow measurement of change over time. For instance, supplements in 1979 were included on immunization, smoking, home health care, eye care, residential mobility, and retirement income. In 1980, the supplements on home health care, residential mobility, and retirement income were continued and a supplement on health insurance was added. In 1981, a child health supplement was included throughout the year. The 1982 NHIS included supplements on health insurance and preventive care. The 1983 NHIS contained questions on alcohol, dental care, physician services, and health insurance. In 1984 the supplement was devoted to health issues of aging; in 1985, health promotion and disease prevention; in 1986, health insurance, dental health, vitamin and mineral intake, longest job worked, and functional limitations; in 1987, cancer risk factors and child adoption; in 1989, mental health. Because of budgetary constraints, beginning in 1985 the supplements have been funded by the agencies requesting the special topics.

With acquired immunodeficiency syndrome (AIDS) reaching epidemic proportions in the United States, and with no cure or vaccine to prevent infection by the virus at this time, a supplement on AIDS knowledge and attitudes was initiated as part of the 1987 NHIS in order to determine the level of knowledge of the U.S. population and to help assess the effectiveness of educational campaigns. This supplement with necessary modifications has been continued throughout 1988, 1989, 1990, and 1991 and will provide continued measurement of the public's knowledge and attitudes about AIDS and changes in these characteristics over time.

National Health and Nutrition Examination Survey

The National Health Survey Act authorized special studies in addition to the continuing household interview survey. Furthermore, the recommendations of the National Committee on Vital and Health Statistics on the subject had also envisioned special studies to include one "to obtain data on undiagnosed and non-manifest diseases" (NCHS, Ser.1, No. 4, 1973). The first Health Examination Survey (HES) was launched in 1959 and was completed in 1962. A traveling staff and mobile examination units were employed for the survey. Data were collected through direct standardized physical examinations, clinical and laboratory tests, and measurements on the total prevalence of certain chronic diseases as well as the distributions of various physical and physiological measures, including blood pressure and serum cholesterol levels. The survey was conducted at two- to four-year cycles through the 1960s.

A decade later the survey was restructured and expanded to include measurements of nutritional status of the population and subsequent monitoring of changes in that status over time. This change reflected the country's and the federal government's shift of emphasis from illness to health maintenance. The survey name was changed to the National Health and Nutrition Examination Survey (NHANES). The first cycle of this expanded survey, NHANES, was initiated in 1970 with data collection beginning in 1971.

To date, five nationwide surveys using health examination procedures have been completed since the inception of this survey program in 1960. In 1982, the survey was directed toward persons of Hispanic origin or descent and was conducted in areas with high concentration of Hispanic population. At the present time, NHANES III is in the field. As with the earlier surveys, NHANES III involves interviews, physical examinations, and biochemical and hematological tests of a representative sample of the U.S. population.

The objectives of both the early HES and the NHANES have been collection of data that can be obtained best or only by direct physical examination, clinical and laboratory tests, and related measurement procedures. Prevalence data are collected for specifically defined diseases or conditions of ill health and normative health-related measurement data are collected that show distributions of the total population with respect to particular parameters, such as blood pressure, visual acuity, and serum cholesterol level.

The sample design for all the HES and NHANES cycles has been multistage, highly clustered probability samples to provide representative national estimates. All of the samples are stratified by broad geographical regions and by population density grouping.

At the present time, NHANES III is in the field. As with the earlier surveys, NHANES III will involve interviews, physical examinations, and biochemical and hematological tests of a representative sample of the U.S. population.

Health Records Survey Program

Soon after the establishment of the National Health Interview Survey and the Health Examination Survey, it became obvious that information on hospitalized illness and injury, out-of-hospital medically attended illness, long-term institutionalized conditions, and data on the use of providers of services and facilities were either not available on a national basis or were inadequate.

As a consequence, by 1960, when the National Health Survey and the National Office of Vital Statistics were combined to form the National Center for Health Statistics, developmental work already had begun for surveys based on records of health facilities and providers of health services.

The Health Records Survey (HRS) program, was conceived originally as one of the three major data collection program activities of the National Health Survey. The surveys under this program were designed to augment the NHIS and NHANES by providing comprehensive statistics on the health of the institutionalized population as well as on the use of all types of health facilities and services.

As stated by NCHS at the time of development of the HRS program, an important distinction between the Health Records Survey program and the other programs of the National Health Survey was that the data are obtained from the provider or facility providing service instead of from the recipient of the service. The rationale for the reliance on the provider, as stated by NCHS, was that providers can have the most accurate and detailed data on diagnosis and treatment, and that providers are a cost-effective source for identifying events such as hospitalization, surgery, and long-term institutionalization, which are relatively rare events in the total population.

The original concept of the HRS encompassed records from all types of medical facilities and institutions, including those from such facilities as hospitals, clinics, dispensaries, physicians' and dentists' offices, and nursing homes. In practice, however, the data are limited to that obtained in the four current surveys: National Hospital Discharge Survey, National Ambulatory Medical Care Survey, National Nursing Home Survey, and the National Master Facility Inventory.

The major part of the data collected is based on existing records. Mechanisms used to obtain the data include abstracts of medical records of institutions, completion of patient encounter forms by physicians, compilation of data from states and professional associations, and purchase of data from private abstract services.

The four component surveys of the HRS, as they have evolved over the years, have provided data for monitoring the supply, organization, and use of health care in specified service setting categories. It is important to note here that these surveys provide data on events or on the characteristics of the provider in a given category. In the 1970s the term Health Records Survey Program was dropped; these surveys began to be referred to as provider surveys and form the basis of the proposed National Health Care Survey, the subject of this study. The four current records, or provider surveys, are described briefly below.

National Master Facility Inventory. As a first order of business to implement the records-based survey program, NCHS developed a current unduplicated list of all facilities for inpatient care in the United States. The National Master Facility Inventory (NMFI) is this list. The NMFI has served as the universe or sampling frame for the health records surveys. Conceptually it includes all types of facilities within scope of the HRS program, with the flexibility to include other types of establishments or health facilities as the program expands. It also serves as a source of statistics on the number, type, and distribution of inpatient facilities in the United States.

The program of the NMFI includes the development and maintenance of a list of names and addresses of all facilities or establishments within its scope and the collection of information that describes them with respect to their size, type, and current status of business. The information not only provides a basis for stratifying the NMFI into homogenous groups for the purpose of sampling designs, but also provides important national statistics about the availability of such facilities nationwide.

The scope of the inventory in its initial stage of development included all hospitals in the United States with 6 or more beds, as well as all resident institutions, except for nursing or personal care homes with less than 3 beds.

Institutions included in the NMFI were establishments that were in business to provide medical, nursing, personal, or custodial care to groups of unrelated individuals who have no usual place of residence elsewhere. Such as:

(1) Establishments that provided nursing care to the aged, infirm, or chronically ill. These included places commonly referred to as nursing homes, homes for the aged, rest homes, boarding homes for the aged, and homes for the needy such as almshouses, county homes, and poor farms. The primary factor that determined if an establishment was in scope was its function of providing some kind of care besides room and board.

(2) Residential schools or homes for the deaf.

(3) Residential schools or homes for the blind.

(4) Homes for unwed mothers.

(5) Orphan asylums and homes for dependent children.

(6) Homes for crippled children.

(7) Homes for incurables.

(8) Residential schools or detention homes for juvenile delinquents.

(9) Prisons, reformatories, and penitentiaries that are operated by the federal or state governments.

The NMFI did not include special dwelling places or group quarters such as hotels, private residential clubs, fraternity or sorority houses, monasteries, nurse's homes, flophouses, or labor camps.

Data items collected in the NMFI included:

- Ownership of the institution,
- Type of services provided,
- Number of beds,
- Number and kinds of staff,
- Patient census,
- Annual number of discharges, and
- Annual number of admissions.

The NMFI has been conducted periodically since 1963. The inventory has been kept current by the periodic addition of names and addresses obtained from state licensing and other agencies for all newly established inpatient facilities. In addition, annual surveys of hospitals and periodic surveys of nursing homes and other facilities are used to update name and location, type of business, number of beds, and number of residents or patients in the facilities and to identify those facilities that have gone out of business.

In the 1970s, all data were obtained through the state statistical agencies participating in the Cooperative Health Statistics System (CHSS). Most of these states, however, had data only on nursing and related care homes. Some of the CHHS states collected data only for nursing homes; NCHS surveyed the other related care homes directly for these states. Hence the scope was limited to data on hospitals and nursing and related care homes. After the elimination of CHHS, NCHS did not go back to collecting data directly from hospitals. Hospital data are purchased from the American Hospital Association and SMG Marketing Group, Inc. In the 1980s the NMFI was once again centralized when the Inventory of Long Term Care Providers was conducted in 1986 (information based on telephone conversations with NCHS staff).

The scope of the 1991 NMFI, renamed the National Health Provider Inventory (NHPI), has been expanded to include information about facilities providing health care, including hospitals, skilled nursing and long-term care units of hospitals, nursing and related care homes, facilities that provide some kind of personal care, board and care or domiciliary care (such as residential care homes, group homes, homes for the aged, family care homes, adult foster care homes, personal care homes, adult congregate living facilities, residential community care facilities, domiciliary care homes), homes for mentally retarded or developmentally disabled people, homes for the mentally ill (such as halfway houses, residential centers for emotionally disturbed children, community residences, and supervised apartments, shelters, and hostels), halfway or quarter-way houses for alcohol or drug abusers, and hospices and home health agencies. Information will be obtained on the certification status under Medicaid or Medicare of the nursing facility, if it is certified under Medicaid as an intermediate care facility for the mentally retarded, and if it is a nursing home unit of a retirement center, as well as the race, sex, and age of residents. The 1991 NHPI will be conducted centrally by the Bureau of the Census as the collecting agent for the NCHS.

National Hospital Discharge Survey. The National Hospital Discharge Survey (NHDS) is a continuing nationwide sample survey of short-stay hospitals in the United States. It has been the principal source of data since 1965 on inpatient use of hospitals by characteristics of patients, expected payment source, length of stay, diagnoses, surgical and nonsurgical procedures, and the patterns of use of care in hospitals of different bed size, ownership type, and geographic region.

The scope of NHDS is limited to discharges from nonfederal hospitals located in the 50 states and the District of Columbia. Only hospitals having 6 or more beds for patient use and an average length of stay for all patients of less than 30 days or those whose specialty is general (medical or surgical), maternity, or children's general are included in the sample.

The NHDS was initiated in fall 1964, the short-stay hospitals listed in the NMFI as of 1964 serving as the sampling frame. The sample was updated periodically with samples of hospitals that opened later. Within each sample hospital, a systematic sample of discharges was selected. Starting in 1985, in addition to manual selection of the sample and transcription of data, NCHS purchased from commercial abstracting services discharge medical abstracts and selected samples from these tapes.

Until 1987 a two-stage stratified sample design was used and the sample was selected from a frame of short-stay hospitals listed in the National Master Facility Inventory. In 1988 when the phased implementation of the National Health Care Survey began, the NHDS was redesigned to incorporate an integrated cluster sample design. A subsample of the NHIS PSUs serves as the sampling frame for NHDS. The redesigned survey includes a three-stage clustered stratified design—the primary sampling units (PSUs), the hospitals within the PSUs, and discharges within hospitals. The redesigned sample contains 542 hospitals, approximately one-third of the sample hospitals providing data through commercial abstract services. In order to ensure continuity of the survey, should a problem arise with the purchase of these data and to provide narrative information for special studies, the design also includes a subsample of 128 hospitals that continue to submit data through the traditional hard copy method of data collection with the

Bureau of the Census or hospital personnel completing the medical abstracts.

The data obtained from the medical abstract form and the abstract service data tapes include:

- Date of birth
- Sex
- Race
- Ethnicity
- Marital status
- Final diagnoses
- Surgical and nonsurgical procedures and dates of procedures
- Expected sources of payment
- Medical record number
- Admission and discharge dates
- Discharge status and disposition
- Residence zip code

The medical record number and patient zip code are confidential information and are not available to the public. Up to seven diagnoses and four procedures are coded for each discharge.

National Ambulatory Medical Care Survey. In the early 1970s the recognition that there was little known on a national basis about medical care provided in physicians' offices that was comparable to information available for hospital care and nursing home care, led to the establishment of the National Ambulatory Medical Care Survey (NAMCS). NAMCS, first fielded in 1973, was designed as a continuing national sample survey to meet the needs and demands for statistical information about the provision of ambulatory medical care services in the United States. Today, however, ambulatory health services are provided in a variety of settings including physicians' offices, health maintenance organizations, and hospital outpatient clinics. Yet NAMCS still is limited to visits to "office-based, patient care, non-federal physicians." As currently designed, it does not include visits to hospital-based physicians; visits to anesthesiologists, pathologists, and radiologists; and visits to physicians who are principally engaged in teaching, research, or administration. Telephone contacts with physicians are also excluded.

The NAMCS was conducted continuously from 1973 through 1981. From 1982 through 1984 the survey was suspended due to budget constraints. The survey was conducted again in 1985. In 1989 survey activities were resumed again on a continuous basis as part of the National Health Care Survey.

During 1973-1985 a multistage probability sample design was used involving samples of PSUs, physician practices within PSUs, and patient visits within physician practices. A modified probability-proportional-to-size sampling procedure using separate sampling frames for metropolitan statistical areas (MSAs) and for nonmetropolitan counties was used to select the first stage sample PSUs independently within each of the four census regions. The second stage consisted of a probability sample of nonfederal, office-based physicians selected from master files maintained by the American Medical Association and the American Osteopathic Association. The third stage is the selection of patient visits within the annual practices of the sample physicians. The 1985 sample included 5,032 physicians and 71,594 patient visits.

In 1989, when the survey was included as a component of the National Health Care Survey, a subsample of the NHIS PSUs was used as the first stage of sample selection. The sample size for the 1989 and 1990 cycles has been reduced by one-half of the 1985 sample size to include 2,500 physicians in office-based practice, with an expected sample of 45,000 patient visits annually. Also, beginning with 1989, data for the survey are being collected annually under an interagency agreement with the Bureau of the Census. Data items for the 1989 and 1990 surveys have remained constant to allow for aggregation over a two-year period.

Data are collected on the characteristics of patients, their diagnoses and symptoms, and on the diagnostic procedures, therapy, drugs prescribed, and payment source associated with each visit to the physician; characteristics of the physician, such as specialty and type of practice.

These data are obtained by means of the induction interview form and patient log and record form. Information is obtained on the physician's specialty, type of practice, and staff. In 1989 questions were included about HMOs and other prepaid programs, on the availability of in-office laboratory testing to provide data on the number of physician offices having in-office laboratory equipment, the nature of in-office tests performed, the degree of quality control exercised in the performance of the tests, and the physicians' knowledge of state testing regulations.

For the 1989-1990 NAMCS, a patient record is completed for each sampled patient visit and contains the following items:

- Patient zip code (new in 1989)
- Date of visit

- Date of birth
- Sex
- Race
- Ethnicity
- Expected source(s) of payment
- New patient
- Referral
- Patient complaint, symptom or reason for visit
- Physician's diagnoses
- Has patient been seen before
- Screening/diagnostic services—includes changes from the 1985 categories, nearly all of which are tests for screening and early detection of disease.
- Medication therapy
- Nonmedication therapy—includes changes from the 1985 categories. New categories include consultation concerning weight reduction, cholesterol reduction, smoking cessation, family planning, and breast self-examination instruction.
- Disposition
- Duration of visit

NCHS plans call for expanding the scope of this survey to cover hospital outpatient and emergency departments beginning in late 1991.

National Nursing Home Survey. The National Nursing Home Survey (NNHS) has been conducted periodically since 1963 and most recently in 1985. Data are collected on a wide range of information about facilities, services provided, staff, financial characteristics, and on residents' personal and health characteristics.

In the 1960s, two surveys of nursing homes were conducted on an ad hoc basis. The need for comprehensive data on a continuing basis became obvious, with the establishment of the Medicaid and Medicare program, increasing use of nursing homes by the elderly population whose numbers were growing, and the overall increasing involvement of the federal government in these and other long-term care issues. In 1973 the National Nursing Home Survey was established in NCHS as a continuing program. The Master Facility Inventory has served as the sampling frame for the surveys.

Subsequent to the two ad hoc surveys in the 1960s, three national nursing home surveys have been conducted. The first national survey was conducted in 1973-1974, the second was conducted in 1977, and the third was conducted in 1985. The next survey is scheduled for 1995.

The 1985 NNHS was a sample survey of nursing and related care homes, their residents, discharges, and staff in the conterminous United States that regularly provide nursing or personal care services to residents, regardless of the level of service provision or the certification status of the facility. Facilities were either free-standing establishments or nursing care units of hospitals, retirement centers, or similar institutions maintaining financial and employee records separate from those of the larger institutions. Residential care facilities were excluded from the scope of the survey, as were those serving only persons with specific health problems, such as mental retardation or alcoholism.

A stratified two-stage probability sample design was used, the first stage being selection of facilities and the second stage being selection of residents, discharges, and registered nurses from the sample facilities.

Data were collected on four major areas:

(1) Facility. Information was obtained by personal interview with the administrator and by mail-back questionnaires. Topics covered included: (1) size, ownership, license and Medicare and Medicaid certification status, number of beds, services offered; (2) staffing patterns including characteristics of registered nurses, work schedule, experience, activities in facility, demographic characteristics, and salary; (3) costs, including total expenses and for major components of operation.

(2) Current residents. Topics covered included: demographic characteristics, activities of daily living, status and living arrangements prior to admission, conditions at admission and at interview, receipt of services, cognitive and emotional status, charges, sources of payment, history of nursing home utilization, and hospitalization during stay.

(3) Discharged residents. Topics covered included: demographic characteristics, history of nursing home utilization, hospitalization during stay, status at discharge, conditions at admission and discharge, sources of payment. Resident information was obtained by personal interview with the nurse who referred to the medical record.

(4) Follow-up. Follow-up information on the two patient samples was collected by means of a computer-assisted telephone interview with a next of kin of the current or discharged resident. The next of kin

interviewed was identified in the current resident and discharged resident questionnaires and included relatives, guardians, and anyone familiar with the sampled resident.

Topics covered included: (1) subject's living arrangements, health, and functional status during the period preceding the admission, (2) history of previous nursing home use activities of daily living, (3) current status and living arrangements, and (4) Medicaid spend-down.

In an attempt to meet the increasing demand for information related to the dynamics of long-term care use, follow-up data were collected in the 1985 NNHS covering a period of one year subsequent to the initial nursing home admission. Since many episodes of alternating institutional, acute hospital, and community care are of considerably longer duration, it became clear that the period of observation needed to be extended. Moreover, data compiled on an event basis do not reveal the interconnections within episodes of illness or utilization or provide information on transitions between hospital, nursing home, and community care. In response to this need, the National Nursing Home Survey Follow-up (NNHS follow-up) was established as a collaborative project between the NCHS and the National Institute on Aging.

The NNHS follow-up is a longitudinal that follows a cohort of surviving current residents and discharged residents sampled from the 1985 NNHS. The primary purpose of the follow-up study is to provide data on the flow of persons in and out of long-term care facilities and hospitals. The study obtains longitudinal information not readily available in the medical record, such as the resident's health and functional status prior to admission, the reason for admission, and a history of previous nursing home admissions, the resident's current functional status, current living arrangements, and nursing home and hospital use subsequent to the last contact and sources of payment.

The NNHS follow-up has initiated three additional contacts with the cohort since the 1985 NNHS. Interviews for all three waves were conducted using a computer-assisted telephone interview (CATI) system. Data collection and data entry are concurrent and computer-controlled.

The first wave of the follow-up was conducted between August and December 1987. The study population consisted of all sampled residents who were still alive, approximately 6,600 subjects. If the subject could not participate, interviews with proxy respondents (primarily next of kin) were conducted. For subjects residing in facilities, administrators or other facility personnel were interviewed.

Wave II of the NNHS follow-up was conducted from July to November 1988, approximately 12 months after the completion of the first wave, and involved approximately 4,000 subjects. The same questionnaire and the CATI system were used for both waves. Respondents were asked about the subject's vital status, living arrangements, and nursing home stays, hospital stays, and sources of payment for stays occurring between the wave I and wave II interviews. For deceased residents the information on cause of death was obtained through the National Death Index.

Interviewing for wave III of the follow-up began the first week of February 1990 and was completed in April 1990. Wave III extends the period of observation for surviving residents in the 1985 NNHS for an additional 18 months and involves approximately 3,000 subjects. The same questionnaire, CATI system, and procedures used in the previous two waves were again applied to wave III. In addition, seven new questions are asked at the end of the interview concerning the disposition of the subject's own home.

Other Related Health Surveys of the Department of Health and Human Services

As stated earlier, many other major data systems are maintained in the other DHHS agencies to meet their special purpose and programmatic needs for statistical information. Some of the major potentially related data systems are briefly described below.

Centers for Disease Control

The Centers for Disease Control (CDC) is the federal agency within the Public Health Service charged with protecting the public health of the nation by providing leadership and direction in the prevention and control of diseases and other preventable conditions and responding to public health emergencies. It is composed of nine major components, one of which is the National Center for Health Statistics.

Behavioral Risk Factor Surveillance System. This surveillance system provides official state health agencies with the funding, training, and consultation necessary to permit them to routinely collect behavioral risk factor information. The data items include weight control, hypertension, physical activity, obesity, mammography, alcohol consumption, seatbelt use, tobacco use, HIV/AIDS, preventive health practices, and routine demographic information such as age, sex, race, and education.

In all, 46 states and jurisdictions participate in this system, which was created in the early 1980s. Each of the states conduct surveys of their noninstitutionalized adult population during the course of the year with 600-3,000 respondents interviewed in each state yearly. Telephone interviewing is employed, and states can add modules of questions to meet special needs. States use the data from this system to develop and evaluate programs and to track progress in reducing behavioral risk factors over time.

Agency for Health Care Policy and Research

The Agency for Health Care Policy and Research was established in 1989 by the Omnibus Budget Reconciliation Act (42 U.S.C. 299) as the successor to the National Center for Health Services Research and Health Care Technology Assessment. The agency is the federal government's focal point for health services research.

National Medical Expenditure Survey. The 1987 National Medical Expenditure Survey (NMES), conducted by the Agency for Health Care Policy and Research, continues a series of national health care expenditures surveys. The last two were conducted in 1980 and 1977. The primary purpose of NMES is to provide the executive branch, the Department of Health and Human Services, and the Congress with national estimates of the use of and expenditures for health care services and of health insurance coverage.

The 1987 NMES is comprised of three components: (1) the Household Survey, (2) an institutional population component that includes the population resident in or admitted to nursing homes and facilities for the mentally retarded over the course of the survey year, and (3) the Survey of American Indians and Alaska Natives (SAIAN), which includes all persons eligible for care through the Indian Health Service and living on or near reservations. Because of the importance of long-term care for the nation's health policy agenda, NMES also provides national estimates on long-term care services and expenditures.

Taken together, the three major components of NMES provide comprehensive, population-based measures of health and functional status, estimates of insurance coverage and of the use of services, expenditures, employment, income, and sources of payment for the calendar year 1987. The long-term care supplement provides estimates of persons with functional disabilities and impairments and their use of formal home and community services, as well as the burden felt by family and friends of providing care.

Although these periodic expenditure surveys provide the most comprehensive data on health expenditures and insurance coverage, they are conducted at infrequent intervals at great cost and are slow to produce accessible data.

Medicare Beneficiary Health Status Registry. A Medicare Beneficiary Health Status Registry (MBHSR) is being developed as a collaborative effort between the Agency for Health Care Policy and Research and the Health Care Financing Administration. The registry is funded by AHCPR and will be implemented by HCFA. It will be a longitudinal database containing information on elderly Medicare beneficiaries obtained by linking health status information from survey data with HCFA's administrative enrollment and utilization files. The survey will gather data on approximately 2 percent of the elderly at the time they enter the Medicare program and at intervals of two to five years thereafter. Data will be gathered of each new Medicare cohort on risk factors, functional status, sociodemographic variables, medical history, and quality of life, thus permitting a projection of their needs. By enrolling successive cohorts over many years, changes in the health and utilization of new entering groups can be monitored over time. Through repeated contacts with the same individuals while they are Medicare beneficiaries, the progression of health and disease can be measured, the relationship between the Medicare program and the health status of its beneficiaries can be examined, and the effectiveness of specific health interventions in influencing the health status of individuals of the group can be evaluated.

The primary goals of the registry are to provide information on measuring the relationship of Medicare-reimbursed services to the health status of Medicare beneficiaries; to describe, analyze, and understand health and disease longitudinally in successive cohorts of Medicare beneficiaries; to describe, analyze, and understand the use and costs of services, long-term utilization patterns, and lifetime Medicare costs of individual cohorts; to monitor access to care in special populations; to assess the effectiveness and impact of specific medical and surgical interventions on the health, quality of life, well-being, and functional status of Medicare beneficiaries; and to monitor existing DHHS "Healthy People 2000" objectives and develop additional ones.

Design and field testing began in September 1990. Implementation is expected in fiscal 1993.

Agency for Alcohol, Drug Abuse, and Mental Health Administration

The Agency for Alcohol, Drug Abuse, and Mental Health Administration (ADAMHA) provides a national focus for the federal effort to increase knowledge and to promote effective strategies in handling health problems and issues associated with the use and abuse of alcohol and drugs and with mental illness and mental health. Its responsibilities include gathering and analyzing data about the extent of alcohol, drug abuse, and mental health problems and the national response to these needs in terms of planning, establishing, and evaluating alcoholism, drug abuse, and mental health programs.

Mental Health Statistics. The National Institute of Mental Health (NIMH) in the Alcohol, Drug Abuse, and Mental Health Administration has been collecting data on inpatient care of the mentally ill in public and private mental hospitals and in psychiatric wards of general hospitals since 1947, when it took over that function from the Bureau of the Census, which had been collecting information on hospitalization of the mentally ill since 1840.

Recognizing that the annual census alone could not provide the range of basic data required on the facilities providing inpatient mental health care, over the years NIMH has taken several steps to correct these shortcomings and, as needs arose, added other types of care settings to the data collection effort and instituted a sample survey program to meet specialized needs.

Today NIMH conducts several inventories of mental health organizations. These data systems are based on questionnaires mailed every other year to mental health organizations in the United States, including psychiatric hospitals, psychiatric services in nonfederal general hospitals, Veterans Administration psychiatric services, residential treatment centers for emotionally disturbed children, freestanding outpatient psychiatric clinics, partial care organizations, and freestanding and multiple care mental health organizations not elsewhere classified.

Information is collected on types of services provided (inpatient, outpatient, and partial care); number of inpatient beds; number of inpatient, outpatient, and partial care additions; average daily and end-of-year inpatient census; patient characteristics; staffing by types of discipline; expenditures; and revenue by source (1983 and 1986 only). Staffing information is collected as of a sample week at the time the inventory is mailed, and information on types of services and beds are collected as of the beginning of the next year.

The sample survey program was initiated in 1969 and today includes admissions to state, county, and private mental hospitals, outpatient psychiatric services, and Veterans Administration psychiatric services. The purpose of these surveys is to obtain data on the sociodemographic, clinical, and treatment characteristics of patients served by these facilities. In general these surveys have been conducted approximately every five years for any specific type of facility. Data are collected on a sample of admissions from a national sample of facilities for one month in the year on age, sex, race, marital status, education, prior psychiatric care, type of services received, and referral on discharge.

The NCHS historically has not gathered data on mental health facilities for their National Master Facility Inventory (NMFI). In the late 1960s, when the expanded and consolidated inventory of mental health organizations was initiated by NIMH, the two agencies reached agreement that NCHS would not collect data on mental health facilities for the NMFI, and NIMH would provide the data collected in their inventory to NCHS for incorporation in the NMFI. These data were then added to the NMFI and reported in the category "other health facilities."

NCHS also has not collected data on the mentally ill on a regular basis in the general health care sector in the same manner that it collects information on general health care. Some information, however, is routinely collected, and other information has been collected on an ad hoc basis if resources are made available by an interested agency. For example:

- The National Hospital Discharge Survey collects information on the mentally ill admitted to short-stay, nonfederal hospitals.

- The National Ambulatory Medical Care Survey collects information on the mentally ill seen in physicians' offices, including psychiatrists' offices. In the 1991 NAMCS a separate item on depression is included in the list of diagnoses instead of relying on physicians to report it.

- The National Nursing Home Survey collects information on mental illness in nursing home residents.

- The National Health and Nutrition Examination Surveys have collected depression data. The NHANES-III, currently in the field, is administering a depression and a manic-depressive instrument.

- The 1989 National Health Interview Survey included a supplement on mental health in collaboration with, and funded by, NIMH. The overall purpose of this supplement was to estimate the number and characteristics of chronically mentally ill persons in the civilian, noninstitutionalized population of the United States. Chronic mental illness is defined by NIMH as "severe and persistent disability resulting primarily from mental illness." It was not the intent of this supplement to estimate the prevalence of any particular disorder.

Alcohol and Drug Abuse Statistics. ADAMHA has instituted several studies to obtain data on the prevalence and trends in alcohol and drug abuse and the treatment facilities. An illustrative few are described below:

The **National Household Survey of Drug Abuse** is a biennial, national sample survey of household population age 12 and older. The survey provides estimates of the lifetime, last year, and current use of marijuana, cigarettes, and alcohol and attitudes about drug abuse. Youths ages 12-17 and young adults ages 18-25 are oversampled, as are blacks and Hispanics. The 1988 survey is the ninth in a series that began in 1971 and is based on personal interviews of a sample of 8,814 persons age 12 and over.

The **National Drug And Alcoholism Treatment Unit Survey** (NDATUS) is a national survey of the scope and use of treatment and prevention services and resources, both privately and publicly funded. This survey is conducted periodically by the National Institute on Drug Abuse and the National Institute on Alcohol Abuse and Alcoholism. Information is obtained from over 12,000 treatment, prevention, and service units on types of services provided, client capacity and census, and funding amounts, as well as client demographic information. Through this survey a National Directory of Drug Abuse and Alcoholism Treatment and Prevention Programs is produced.

The **Sample Survey of NDATUS Clients** will be a sample survey of clients drawn from a representative sample of the drug abuse and alcohol treatment units. The study will provide for the first time data on information on the characteristics of alcohol and drug abuse treatment programs and on types and duration of treatment and collateral client-focused activities. Client characteristics will include previous treatment history, diagnostic data about drug and alcohol use, amount, patterns, and related impairments. Clients will be reinterviewed at 3 and 15 months to determine subsequent treatment and changes in use and impairments.

Prevalence and Impact of Alcohol and Drug Abuse Dependence in Short-term General Hospitals will be a one-time study to determine the national prevalence rates of alcohol abuse and alcoholism and polysubstance abuse in short-term, general, nonfederal hospitals; it will also determine the impact of alcohol and other drug abuse and dependencies on hospital resource utilization, charges, and costs.

Drug Abuse Warning Network (DAWN) is a large-scale ongoing drug abuse data collection system based on information from a nonrandom sample of emergency room and medical examiner facilities. DAWN collects information only about those drug abuse occurrences that have resulted in a medical crisis or death. Major objectives include the monitoring of patterns and trends of drug abuse, identification of substances associated with drug abuse episodes, and the assessment of drug-related consequences and other health hazards.

Health Care Financing Administration

The Health Care Financing Administration (HCFA) was established in 1977, placing under one administration the oversight of the Medicare and Medicaid programs and related federal medical care quality control staffs.
HCFA maintains a comprehensive system of administrative data on Medicare

enrollment, use, diagnosis, provider characteristics, costs, charges, and payments based on the claims payment files. Administrative data systems, of course, are a by-product of program administration. Although they have many potential uses, they cannot tell us, for example, about services currently not covered by Medicare but that may be likely targets of new legislation, or about sources of payment other than Medicare, people who do not use Medicare services, or characteristics of beneficiaries that determine their use of services and costs.

HCFA has taken several steps to enhance the usefulness of its data by developing systems to obtain information about the health status and sociodemographic variables of the beneficiaries that can be linked to the administrative files for analysis. Some of these databases are described below.

Medicare Current Beneficiary Survey. The Medicare Current Beneficiary Survey (MCBS), developed by the Health Care Financing Administration, is designed to be an ongoing multipurpose survey for use by all components of HCFA, the department, and others concerned with Medicare policy. The MCBS is focused on health care use and expenditure in the Medicare population and determinants thereof, issues that are of prime importance to HCFA.

The core of the MCBS is a series of interviews of a representative sample of the Medicare population to obtain information on their patterns of health service use and cost over time, sources of coverage and payment, assets and income, demographic characteristics, health and functional status, health and work history, and family supports. The same people will be interviewed three times a year over several years to observe changes in use with changes in coverage, and to observe processes that occur over time, such as institutionalization or spending down of assets. The survey will produce data sets suitable for both longitudinal and cross-sectional analysis.

In addition to the core items, periodic or one-time supplements will be included in each of the three annual rounds. These will collect information on relatively stable characteristics of the respondents such as work history, or on special topics of current policy interest to HCFA, such as access to care or perceptions about health maintenance organizations. They may also contain questions that need not be asked each time but may be asked annually, such as income and assets.

The MCBS sample will consist of 12,000 individuals sampled from the Medicare Enrollment File to be representative of the Medicare population as a whole and by age group, enrollment type (aged or disabled), urban or rural residence, and among the aged, whether or not institutionalized. The sample will be adjusted annually for attrition, as well as for newly eligible persons.

Survey data files will be matched to HCFA claims payment and other administrative records such as the National Death Index, Social Security records, and the Area Resource File. Pilot testing of all forms and procedures has been completed and data collection is under way.

Nursing Home Quality Assessment. The Omnibus Reconciliation Act of 1987 requires that each resident of a Medicare or Medicaid certified nursing facility have a periodic standardized, accurate, and reproducible comprehensive assessment of his or her functional capacity using a Resident Assessment Instrument (RAI) specified by the state. In addition, the instrument must include a uniform minimum data set of core elements, common definitions, and utilization guidelines specified by HCFA.

According to HCFA plans, implementation will be phased in so that initially the RAI will be administered only for new admissions. Reassessments will be conducted when significant changes in the patient's status have occurred. The database generated from the RAI over time has the potential for being used for research purposes in addition to the administrative uses for which the instrument was originally developed, which raises concerns about the quality and reliability of the data.

Medicare Provider Analysis and Review—Medicare Stay Records. An Inpatient Hospital Stay Record containing information about a person's stay in a hospital from admission through discharge is created for 100 percent of Medicare enrollees. Stay records are used to compile many health insurance utilization tables and the Medicare Provider Analysis and Review (MEDPAR) files. This record contains use information from bills, demographic information about the enrollee, and provider characteristics data. Stay records are also prepared for stays in skilled nursing facilities (SNF). The SNF stay record is essentially the same as the hospital record.

Part B Medicare Annual Data System. The Part B Medicare Annual Data System (BMAD) system collects information in each carrier's history of claims processed. The data are produced and submitted from the Medicare claims history for the preceding year and are submitted annually. The Part B data are provided in four separate files: (1) The Procedures File—provides an array of every procedure processed showing the relative frequency, submitted charge, and paid amounts. This file gives HCFA detail on all the services processed by Medicare carriers. (2) The Prevailing Charge File—supplies HCFA with the prevailing charge limits for every procedure shown on a carrier's procedure file submittal. It allows HCFA to study and accurately project payment levels. (3) The Provider File—contains line-by-line detail from claims history of procedures rendered by a 1-percent sample of physician suppliers. These data allow HCFA to study the impact of actual and physicians' projected program changes on the suppliers. (4) The Beneficiary File—this is a 5-percent beneficiary history sample file. It contains the detailed claims history of procedures received by the sample beneficiaries. This file also collects the claims detail for all End Stage Renal Disease (ESRD) beneficiaries. This file allows HCFA to link, based on the health insurance claims number, a beneficiary's Part A and Part B service utilization data.

CONCLUSION

The brief descriptions presented above of only some of the national health data systems maintained by the federal government provide a clear illustration of a large number of statistical activities in place and new ones being developed. Despite these various activities, we still lack important statistical information needed for monitoring and evaluating the important changes occurring in the availability, financing, and delivery of health care. The need for these data will become even more critical in the years to come, as the country debates and attempts to reach informed decisions on major health care reform, an issue that will be on the forefront for the next several years in the federal government, the professional community, and the public.

APPENDIX D

Statutory Authorities

The National Health Survey Act
The National Center for Health Statistics

APPENDIX II

NATIONAL HEALTH SURVEY ACT

PUBLIC LAW 652 - 84TH CONGRESS

CHAPTER 510 - 2D SESSION-S. 3076

AN ACT

To provide for a continuing survey and special studies of sickness and disability in the United States, and for periodic reports of the results thereof, and for other purposes.

Be it enacted by the Senate and House of Representatives of the United States of America in Congress assembled, That this Act may be cited as the "National Health Survey Act".

Sec. 2. (a) The Congress hereby finds and declares—

(1) that the latest information on the number and relevant characteristics of persons in the country suffering from heart disease, cancer, diabetes, arthritis and rheumatism, and other diseases, injuries, and handicapping conditions is now seriously out of date; and

(2) that periodic inventories providing reasonably current information on these matters are urgently needed for purposes such as (A) appraisal of the true state of health of our population (including both adults and children), (B) adequate planning of any programs to improve their health, (C) research in the field of chronic diseases, and (D) measurement of the numbers of persons in the working ages so disabled as to be unable to perform gainful work.

(b) It is, therefore, the purpose of this Act to provide (1) for a continuing survey and special studies to secure on a non-compulsory basis accurate and current statistical information on the amount, distribution, and effects of illness and disability in the United States and the services received for or because of such conditions; and (2) for studying methods and survey techniques for securing such statistical information, with a view toward their continuing improvement.

Sec. 3. Part A of title III of the Public Health Service Act (42 U. S. C. ch. 6A) is amended by adding after section 304 the following new section:

"NATIONAL HEALTH SURVEYS AND STUDIES

Sec. 305. (a) The Surgeon General is authorized (1) to make, by sampling or other appropriate means, surveys and special studies of the population of the United States to determine the extent of illness and disability and related information such as: (A) the number, age, sex, ability to work or engage in other activities, and occupation or activities of persons afflicted with chronic or other disease or injury or handicapping condition; (B) the type of disease or injury or handicapping condition of each person so afflicted; (C) the length of time that each such person has been prevented from carrying on his occupation or activities; (D) the amounts and types of services received for or because of such conditions; and (E) the economic and other impacts of such conditions; and (2) in connection therewith, to develop and test new or improved methods for obtaining current data on illness and disability and related information.

"(b) The Surgeon General is authorized, at appropriate intervals, to make available, through publications and otherwise, to any interested governmental or other public or private agencies, organizations, or groups, or to the public, the results of surveys or studies made pursuant to subsection (a).

"(c) For each fiscal year beginning after June 30, 1956, there are authorized to be appropriated such sums as the Congress may determine for carrying out the provisions of this section.

"(d) To assist in carrying out the provisions of this section the Surgeon General is authorized and directed to cooperate and consult with the Departments of Commerce and Labor and any other interested Federal Departments or agencies and with State health departments. For such purpose he shall utilize insofar as possible the services or facilities of any agency of the Federal Government and, without regard to section 3709 of the Revised Statutes, as amended, of any appropriate State or other public agency, and may, without regard to section 3709 of the Revised Statutes, as amended, utilize the services or facilities of any private agency, organization, group, or individual, in accordance with written agreements between the head of such agency, organization, or group, or such individual, and the Secretary of Health, Education, and Welfare. Payment, if any, for such services or facilities shall be made in such amounts as may be provided in such agreement."

Sec. 4. Section 301 of the Public Health Service Act (42 U. S. C. 241) is amended by striking out the word "and" at the end of paragraph (f), redesignating paragraph (g) as paragraph (h), and inserting immediately following paragraph (f) the following new paragraph:

"(g) Make available, to health officials, scientists, and appropriate public and other nonprofit institutions and organizations, technical advice and assistance on the application of statistical methods to experiments, studies, and surveys in health and medical fields: and".

Approved July 3, 1956.

Excerpts from the Public Health Service Act

General authority respecting research, evaluations, and demonstrations in health statistics, health services, and health care technology assessment

Sec. 304 [242b] (a) The Secretary may, through the Agency for Health Care Policy and Research or the National Center for Health Statistics or using National Research Service Awards or other appropriate authorities, undertake and support training programs to provide for an expanded and continuing supply of individuals qualified to perform the research, evaluation, and demonstration projects set forth in section 306 and in title IX.

(b) To implement subsection (a), and section 306, the Secretary may, in addition to any other authority which under other provisions of this Act or any other law may be used by him to implement such subsection, do the following:

(1) Utilize personnel and equipment, facilities, and other physical resources of the Department of Health and Human Services, permit appropriate (as determined by the Secretary) entities and individuals to utilize the physical resources of such Department, provide technical assistance and advice, make grants to public and nonprofit private entities and individuals, and, when appropriate, enter into contracts with public and private entities and individuals.

(2) Admit and treat at hospitals and other facilities of the Service persons not otherwise eligible for admission and treatment at such facilities.

(3) Secure, from time to time and for such periods as the Secretary deems advisable but in accordance with section 3109 of title 5, United States Code, the assistance and advice of consultants from the United States or abroad. The Secretary may for the purpose of carrying out the functions set forth in sections 305, 306, and 309, obtain (in accordance with section 3109 of title 5 of the United States Code, but without regard to the limitation in such section on the number of days or the period of service) for each of the centers the services of not more than fifteen experts who have appropriate scientific or professional qualifications.

(4) Acquire, construct, improve, repair, operate, and maintain laboratory, research, and other necessary facilities and equipment, and such other real or personal property (including patents) as the Secretary deems necessary; and acquire, without regard to the Act of March 3, 1877 (40 U.S.C. 34), by lease or otherwise, through the Administrator of General Services, buildings or parts of buildings in the District of Columbia or communities located adjacent to the District of Columbia.

(c)(1) The Secretary shall coordinate all health services research, evaluations, and demonstrations, all health statistical and epidemiological activities, and all research, evaluations, and demonstrations respecting the assessment of health care technology undertaken and supported through units of the Department of Health and Human Services. To the maximum extent feasible such coordination shall be carried out through the Agency for Health Care Policy and Research and the National Center for Health Statistics.

(2) The Secretary shall coordinate the health services research, evaluations, and demonstrations, the health statistical and (where appropriate) epidemiological activities, and the research, evaluations, and demonstrations respecting the assessment of health care technology authorized by this Act through the Agency for Health Care Policy and Research and the National Center for Health Statistics.

(d)(1) The Secretary, with the advice and assistance of the National Academy of Sciences (acting through the Institute of Medicine and other appropriate units), shall, in cooperation with the Administrator of the Environmental Protection Agency, the Secretary of Labor, the Consumer Product Safety Commission, the Council of Economic Advisers, the Council on Wage and Price Stability, the Council on Environmental Quality, and other entities of the Federal Government which the Secretary determines have the expertise in the subject of the study prescribed by this paragraph, conduct, with funds appropriated under section 308(i)(2), an ongoing study of the present and projected future health costs of pollution and other environmental conditions resulting from human activity (including human activity in any place in the indoor or outdoor environment, including places of employment and residence). In conducting the study, the Secretary shall, to the extent feasible—

(A) identify the pollution (and the pollutants responsible for the pollution) and other environmental conditions which are, or may reasonably be anticipated to be, responsible for causing, contributing to, increasing susceptibility to, or aggravating human diseases and adverse effects on humans;

(B) identify each such disease and adverse effect on humans and specifically determine whether cancer, birth defects, genetic damage, emphysema, asthma, bronchitis, and other respiratory diseases, heart disease, stroke, and mental illness and impairment are such a disease or effect;

(C) identify (on a national, regional, or other geographical basis) the source or sources of such pollutants and conditions and estimate the portion of each pollutant and the extent of each condition which can be traced to a specific type of source;

(D) ascertain (i) the extent to which the pollutants and conditions identified under subparagraph (A) are, or may reasonably be anticipated to be, responsible, individually or collectively, for causing, contributing to, increasing susceptibility to, or aggravating the diseases and effects identified under subparagraph (B), and (ii) the effect upon the incidence or severity of specific diseases and effects of individual or collective, as appropriate, incremental reductions in the pollutants and changes in such conditions; and

(E) quantify (i) the present and projected future health costs of the diseases and effects identified under subparagraph (B), and (ii) the reduction in health costs which would result from each incremental reduction and change referred to in subparagraph (D)(ii).

(2) The Secretary shall enter into appropriate arrangements with the Academy under which the Secretary shall be responsible for expenses incurred by the Academy in connection with the study prescribed by paragraph (1).

(3) The first report on the study prescribed by paragraph (1) shall be made to the Committee on Human Resources of the Senate and the Committee on Energy and Commerce of the House of Representatives by the Secretary not later than eighteen

months after the date of the enactment of this subsection. Subsequent reports on the study shall be made by the Secretary every three years after the date the first report is submitted. Each report shall (A) identify deficiencies and limitations in the data on the matters considered in the study and recommend actions which may be taken to eliminate such deficiencies and limitations, (B) include such recommendations for legislation as the Secretary determines appropriate, (C) include recommendations for facilitating studies of the effects of hazardous substances on humans, and (D) include a description of any administrative action proposed to be taken by the Secretary, the Administrator of the Environmental Protection Agency, the Secretary of Labor, and the Consumer Product Safety Commission to reduce the costs which have been quantified under paragraph (1)(E)(i). In conducting the study, the Secretary shall seek assistance from public and private health financing entities in securing the data needed for the study.

(4) For purposes of paragraph (1), the term "health costs of pollution and other environmental conditions" means the costs of human diseases and other adverse effects on humans which pollution and other environmental conditions are, or may reasonably be anticipated to be, responsible for causing, contributing to, increasing susceptibility to, or aggravating, including the costs of preventing such diseases and effects, the costs of the treatment, cure, convalescence, and rehabilitation of persons afflicted by such diseases, costs reasonably attributable to pain and suffering from such diseases and effects, loss of income and future earnings resulting from such diseases and effects, adverse effects on productivity (and thus increases in production costs and consumer prices) resulting from such diseases and effects, loss of tax revenues resulting from such decreases in earnings and productivity, costs to the welfare and unemployment compensation systems and the programs of health benefits under titles XVIII and XIX of the Social Security Act resulting from such diseases and effects, the overall increases in costs throughout the economy resulting from such diseases and effects, and other related direct and indirect costs.

National Center for Health Statistics

Sec. 306 [242k] (a) There is established in the Department of Health and Human Services the National Center for Health Statistics (hereinafter in this section referred to as the "Center") which shall be under the direction of a Director who shall be appointed by the Secretary. The Secretary, acting through the Center, shall conduct and support statistical and epidemiological activities for the purpose of improving the effectiveness, efficiency, and quality of health services in the United States.

(b) In carrying out subsection (a), the Secretary, acting through the Center—
(1) shall collect statistics on—
(A) the extent and nature of illness and disability of the population of the United States (or of any groupings of the people included in the population), including life expectancy, the incidence of various acute and chronic illnesses, and infant and maternal morbidity and mortality,
(B) the impact of illness and disability of the population on the economy of the United States and on other aspects of the well-being of its population (or of such groupings),
(C) environmental, social, and other health hazards,
(D) determinants of health,
(E) health resources, including physicians, dentists, nurses, and other health professionals by specialty and type of practice and the supply of

services by hospitals, extended care facilities, home health agencies, and other health institutions,

(F) utilization of health care, including utilization of (i) ambulatory health services by specialties and types of practice of the health professionals providing such services, and (ii) services of hospitals, extended care facilities, home health agencies, and other institutions,

(G) health care costs and financing, including the trends in health care prices and cost, the sources of payments for health care services, and Federal, State, and local governmental expenditures for health care services, and

(H) family formation, growth, and dissolution;

(2) shall undertake and support (by grant or contract) research, demonstrations, and evaluations respecting new or improved methods for obtaining current data on the matters referred to in paragraph (1);

(3) may undertake and support (by grant or contract) epidemiological research, demonstrations, and evaluations on the matters referred to in paragraph (1); and

(4) may collect, furnish, tabulate, and analyze statistics, and prepare studies on matters referred to in paragraph (1) upon request of public and nonprofit private entities under arrangements under which the entities will pay the cost of the service provided.

Amounts appropriated to the Secretary from payments made under arrangements made under paragraph (4) shall be available to the Secretary for obligation until expended.

(c) The Center shall furnish such special statistical and epidemiological compilations and surveys as the Committee on Human Resources and the Committee on Appropriations of the Senate and the Committee on Energy and Commerce and the Committee on Appropriations of the House of Representatives may request. Such statistical and epidemiological compilations and surveys shall not be made subject to the payment of the actual or estimated cost of the preparation of such compilations and surveys.

(d) To insure comparability and reliability of health statistics, the Secretary shall, through the Center, provide adequate technical assistance to assist State and local jurisdictions in the development of model laws dealing with issues of confidentiality and comparability of data.

(e) For the purpose of producing comparable and uniform health information and statistics, there is established the Cooperative Health Statistics System. The Secretary, acting through the Center, shall—

(1) coordinate the activities of Federal agencies involved in the design and implementation of the System;

(2) undertake and support (by grant or contract) research, development, demonstrations, and evaluations respecting the System;

(3) make grants to and enter into contracts with State and local health agencies to assist them in meeting the costs of data collection and other activities carried out under the System; and

(4) review the statistical activities of the Department of Health and Human Services to assure that they are consistent with the System.

States participating in the System shall designate a State agency to administer or be responsible for the administration of the statistical activities within the State under the System. The Secretary, acting through the Center, shall prescribe guidelines to assure that statistical activities within States participating in the System produce uniform and timely data and assure appropriate access to such data.

(f) To assist in carrying out this section, the Secretary, acting through the Center, shall cooperate and consult with the Departments of Commerce and Labor and any other interested Federal departments or agencies and with State and local health departments and agencies. For such purpose he shall utilize insofar as possible the services or facilities of any agency of the Federal Government and, without regard to section 3709 of the Revised Statutes (41 U.S.C. 5), of any appropriate State or other public agency, and may, without regard to such section, utilize the services or facilities of any private agency, organization, group, or individual, in accordance with written agreements between the head of such agency, organization, or group and the Secretary or between such individual and the Secretary. Payment, if any, for such services or facilities shall be made in such amounts as may be provided in such agreement.

(g) To secure uniformity in the registration and collection of mortality, morbidity, and other health data, the Secretary shall prepare and distribute suitable and necessary forms for the collection and compilation of such data which shall be published as a part of the health reports published by the Secretary.

(h)(1) There shall be an annual collection of data from the records of births, deaths, marriages, and divorces in registration areas. The data shall be obtained only from and restricted to such records of the States and municipalities which the Secretary, in his discretion, determines possess records affording satisfactory data in necessary detail and form. The Secretary shall encourage States and registration areas to obtain detailed data on ethnic and racial populations, including subpopulations of Hispanics, Asian Americans, and Pacific Islanders with significant representation in the State or registration area. Each State or registration area shall be paid by the Secretary the Federal share of its reasonable costs (as determined by the Secretary) for collecting and transcribing (at the request of the Secretary and by whatever method authorized by him) its records for such data.

(2) There shall be an annual collection of data from a statistically valid sample concerning the general health, illness, and disability status of the civilian noninstitutionalized population. Specific topics to be addressed under this paragraph, on an annual or periodic basis, shall include the incidence of illness and accidental injuries, prevalence of chronic diseases and impairments, disability, physician visits, hospitalizations, and the relationship between demographic and socioeconomic characteristics and health characteristics.

(i) The Center may provide to public and nonprofit private entities engaged in health planning activities technical assistance in the effective use in such activities of statistics collected or compiled by the Center.

(j) In carrying out the requirements of section 304(c) and paragraph (1) of subsection (e) of this section, the Secretary shall coordinate health statistical and epidemiological activities of the Department of Health and Human Services by—

(1) establishing standardized means for the collection of health information and statistics under laws administered by the Secretary;

(2) developing, in consultation with the National Committee on Vital and Health Statistics, and maintaining the minimum sets of data needed on a continuing basis to fulfill the collection requirements of subsection (b)(1);

(3) after consultation with the National Committee on Vital and Health Statistics, establishing standards to assure the quality of health statistical and epidemiological data collection, processing, and analysis;

(4) in the case of proposed health data collections of the Department which are required to be reviewed by the Director of the Office of Management and Budget under section 3509 of title 44, United States Code, reviewing such proposed collections to determine whether they conform with the minimum sets of data and the standards promulgated pursuant to paragraphs (2) and (3), and if any such proposed collection is found not to be in conformance, by taking such action as may be necessary to assure that it will conform to such sets of data and standards, and

(5) periodically reviewing ongoing health data collections of the Department, subject to review under such section 3509, to determine if the collections are being conducted in accordance with the minimum sets of data and the standards promulgated pursuant to paragraphs (2) and (3) and, if any such collection is found not to be in conformance, by taking such action as may be necessary to assure that the collection will conform to such sets of data and standards not later than the nineteenth day after the date of the completion of the review of the collection.

(k)(1) There is established in the Office of the Secretary a committee to be known as the National Committee on Vital and Health Statistics (hereinafter in this subsection, referred to as the "Committee") which shall consist of 16 members.

(2)(A) The members of the Committee shall be appointed by the Secretary from among persons who have distinguished themselves in the fields of health statistics, health planning, epidemiology, and the provision of health services. Except as provided in subparagraph (B), members of the Committee shall be appointed for terms of 4 years.

(B)(i) In the case of membership terms on the Committee under this subsection (as in effect prior to January 1, 1988) that expire in calendar year 1988, the appointments to three such terms in such calendar year shall be for a period of 4 years and the appointments to two such terms in such calendar year shall be for a period of 3 years, as designated by the Secretary.

(ii) In the case of membership terms on the Committee under this subsection (as in effect prior to January 1, 1988) that expire in calendar year 1989, one such term shall be extended for an additional consecutive 1-year period, as designated by the Secretary.

(iii) In the case of membership terms on the Committee under this subsection (as in effect prior to January 1, 1988) that expire in calendar year 1990, two of such terms shall each be extended for an additional consecutive 1-year period, as designated by the Secretary.

(3) Members of the Committee shall be compensated in accordance with section 208(c).

(4) It shall be the function of the Committee to assist and advise the Secretary—

(A) to delineate statistical problems bearing on health and health services which are of national or international interest;

(B) to stimulate studies of such problems by other organizations and agencies whenever possible or to make investigations of such problems through subcommittees;

(C) to determine, approve, and revise the terms, definitions, classifications, and guidelines for assessing health status and health services, their distribution and costs, for use (i) within the Department of Health and Human Services, (ii) by all programs administered or funded by the Secretary, including the Federal-State-local cooperative health statistics system referred to in subsection (e), and (iii) to the extent possible as determined by the head of the agency involved, by the Veterans' Administration, the Department of Defense, and other Federal agencies concerned with health and health services;

(D) with respect to the design of and approval of health statistical and health information systems concerned with the collection, processing, and tabulation of health statistics within the Department of Health and Human Services, with respect to the Cooperative Health Statistics System established under subsection (e), and with respect to the standardized means for the collection of health information and statistics to be established by the Secretary under subsection (j)(1);

(E) to review and comment on findings and proposals developed by other organizations and agencies and to make recommendations for their adoption or implementation by local, State, national, or international agencies;

(F) to cooperate with national committees of other countries and with the World Health Organization and other national agencies in the studies of problems of mutual interest; and

(G) to issue an annual report on the state of the Nation's health, its health services, their costs and distributions, and to make proposals for improvement of the Nation's health statistics and health information systems.

(5) In carrying out health statistical activities under this part, the Secretary shall consult with, and seek the advice of, the Committee and other appropriate professional advisory groups.

(l)(1) The Secretary, acting through the Center, shall develop a plan for the collection and coordination of statistical and epidemiological data on the effects of the environment on health. Such plan shall include a review of the data now available on health effects, deficiencies in such data, and methods by which existing data deficiencies can be corrected. The Secretary shall submit such plan to the Congress not later than January 1, 1980.

(2)(A) The Secretary, acting through the Center and in cooperation with the Office of Federal Statistical Policy and Standards, shall establish, not later than two years after the date of the enactment of this subsection, guidelines for the collection, compilation, analysis, publication, and distribution of statistics and information necessary for determining the effects of conditions of employment and indoor and outdoor environmental conditions on the public health. Guidelines established under this subparagraph shall not (i) authorize or require the disclosure of any matter described in section 552(b)(6) of title 5, United States Code, and (ii) authorize or require the disclosure of any statistics or other information which is exempt from disclosure pursuant to subsection (a) of section 552 of title 5, United States Code, by reason of subsection (b)(4) of such section. The guidelines shall be reviewed and, if appropriate, revised at least every three years after the date they are initially established. Guidelines shall take effect on the date of the promulgation of the regulation establishing or revising the guidelines or such later date as may be specified in the guidelines.

(B) The guidelines shall be designed —

(i) to improve coordination of environmental and health studies, statistics, and information, and to prevent overlap and unnecessary duplication with respect to such studies, statistics, and information;

(ii) to assure that such studies, statistics, and information will be available to executive departments responsible for the administration of laws relating to the protection of the public health and safety or the environment;

(iii) to encourage the more effective use of executive departments of such studies, statistics, and information;

(iv) to improve the statistical validity and reliability of such studies, statistics, and information; and

(v) to assure greater responsiveness by the Department of Health and Human Services and other executive departments in meeting informational and analytical needs for determining the effects of employment and indoor and outdoor environmental conditions on public health.

(C) In establishing and revising guidelines under subparagraph (A), the Secretary shall take into consideration the plan developed pursuant to paragraph (1).

(D)(i) Each executive department shall comply with the substantive and procedural requirements of the guidelines.

(ii) The President shall by Executive order require each executive department to comply with requests, made in accordance with the guidelines, by the Secretary, the Administrator of the Environmental Protection Agency, the Consumer Product Safety Commission, or the Secretary of Labor for statistics and information.

(iii) The President may by Executive order exempt any executive department from compliance with a requirement of the guidelines respecting specific statistics or other information if the President determines that the exemption is necessary in the interest of national security.

(E) In carrying out his duties under this paragraph, the Secretary, acting through the Center, shall, insofar as practicable, provide for coordination of his activities with those of other Federal agencies and interagency task forces relating to the collection, analysis, publication, or distribution of statistics and information necessary for determining the effects of conditions of employment and indoor and outdoor environmental conditions on the public health.

(F) For purposes of this paragraph, the term "guidelines" means the guidelines, either as initially established or as revised, in effect under this paragraph.

(3) The Secretary, acting through the Center, shall conduct a study of the issues respecting, and the recommendations for, establishing a Federal system to assist, in a manner designed to avoid invasion of personal privacy, Federal, State, and other entities in locating individuals who have been or may have been exposed to hazardous substances to determine the effect on their health of such exposure and to assist them in obtaining appropriate medical care and treatment. In conducting such study, the Secretary may consult with any public and private entity which it determines has expertise on any matter to be considered in the study. Not later than one year after the date of the enactment of this subsection, the Secretary shall complete the study and report to the Congress the results of the study and any recommendations for legislation or administrative action.

(4) In carrying out paragraphs (1), (2), and (3), the Secretary shall consult with and take into consideration any recommendations of the Task Force on Environmental Cancer and Heart and Lung Disease, the Administrator of the Environmental Protection Agency, the Secretary of Labor, the Consumer Product Safety Commission, the Council on Environmental Quality, the National Committee on Vital and Health Statistics, and the National Academy of Sciences (including the Institute of Medicine and any other unit of the Academy).

(m) In carrying out this section, the Secretary, acting through the Center, shall collect and analyze adequate health data that is specific to particular ethnic and racial populations, including data collected under national health surveys. Activities carried out under this subsection shall be in addition to any activities carried out under subsection (n).

(n)(1) The Secretary, acting through the Center, may make grants to public and nonprofit private entities for—

(A) the conduct of special surveys or studies on the health of ethnic and racial populations or subpopulations;

(B) analysis of data on ethnic and racial populations and subpopulations; and

(C) research on improving methods for developing statistics on ethnic and racial populations and subpopulations.

(2) The Secretary, acting through the Center, may provide technical assistance, standards, and methodologies to grantees supported by this subsection in order to maximize the data quality and comparability with other studies.

(3) Provisions of section 308 (d) do not apply to surveys or studies conducted by grantees under this subsection unless the Secretary, in accordance with regulations the Secretary may issue, determines that such provisions are necessary for the conduct of the survey or study and receives adequate assurance that the grantee will enforce such provisions.

(o)(1) For health statistical and epidemiological activities undertaken or supported under subsections (a) through (m), there are authorized to be appropriated such sums as may be necessary for each of the fiscal years 1991 through 1993.

(2) For activities authorized in subsection (n), there are authorized to be appropriated $5,000,000 for fiscal year 1991, $7,500,000 for fiscal year 1992, and $10,000,000 for fiscal year 1993. Of such amounts, the Secretary shall use not more than 10 percent for administration and for activities described in subsection (n)(2).

International cooperation

Sec. 307 [242l] (a) For the purpose of advancing the status of the health sciences in the United States (and thereby the health of the American people), the Secretary may participate with other countries in cooperative endeavors in biomedical research, health care technology, and the health services research and statistical activities authorized by section 306 and by title IX.

(b) In connection with the cooperative endeavors authorized by subsection (a), the Secretary may—

(1) make such use of resources offered by participating foreign countries as he may find necessary and appropriate;

(2) establish and maintain fellowships in the United States and in participating foreign countries;

(3) make grants to public institutions or agencies and to nonprofit private institutions or agencies in the United States and in participating foreign countries for the purpose of establishing and maintaining the fellowships authorized by paragraph (2);

(4) make grants or loans of equipment and materials, for use by public or nonprofit private institutions or agencies, or by individuals, in participating foreign countries;

(5) participate and otherwise cooperate in any international meetings, conferences, or other activities concerned with biomedical research, health services research, health statistics, or health care technology;

(6) facilitate the interchange between the United States and participating foreign countries, and among participating foreign countries, of research scientists and experts who are engaged in experiments or programs of biomedical research, health services research, health statistical activities, or health care

technology activities, and in carrying out such purpose may pay per diem compensation, subsistence, and travel for such scientists and experts when away from their places of residence at rates not to exceed those provided in section 5703(b) of title 5, United States Code, for persons in the Government service employed intermittently; and

(7) procure, in accordance with section 3109 of title 5, United States Code, the temporary or intermittent services of experts or consultants.

The Secretary may not, in the exercise of his authority under this section, provide financial assistance for the construction of any facility in any foreign country.

General provisions respecting effectiveness, efficiency, and quality of health services

Sec. 308 [242m] (a)(1) Not later than March 15 of each year, the Secretary shall submit to the President and Congress the following reports:

(A) A report on—
  (i) the administration of sections 304, 306, and 307 and title IX during the preceding fiscal year; and
  (ii) the current state and progress of health services research, health statistics, and health care technology.

(B) A report on health care costs and financing. Such report shall include a description and analysis of the statistics collected under section 306(b)(1)(G).

(C) A report on health resources. Such report shall include a description and analysis, by geographical area, of the statistics collected under section 306(b)(1)(E).

(D) A report on the utilization of health resources. Such report shall include a description and analysis, by age, sex, income, and geographic area, of the statistics collected under section 306(b)(1)(F).

(E) A report on the health of the Nation's people. Such report shall include a description and analysis, by age, sex, income, and geographic area, of the statistics collected under section 306(b)(1)(A).

(2) The reports required by subparagraphs (B) through (E) of paragraph (2) shall be prepared through the Agency for Health Care Policy and Research and the National Center for Health Statistics.

(3) The Office of Management and Budget may review any report required by paragraph (1) of this subsection before its submission to Congress, but the Office may not revise any such report or delay its submission beyond the date prescribed for its submission, and may submit to Congress its comments respecting any such report.

(b)(1) No grant or contract may be made under section 304, 306, or 307, unless an application therefor has been submitted to the Secretary in such form and manner, and containing such information, as the Secretary may by regulation prescribe and unless a peer review group referred to in paragraph (2) has recommended the application for approval.

(2)(A) Each application submitted for a grant or contract under section 306 in an amount exceeding $50,000 of direct costs and for a health services research, evaluation, or demonstration project, or for a grant under section 306(n), shall be submitted to a peer review group for an evaluation of the technical and scientific merits of the proposals made in each such application. The Director of the National

Center for Health Statistics shall establish such peer review groups as may be necessary to provide for such an evaluation of each such application.

(B) A peer review group to which an application is submitted pursuant to subparagraph (A) shall report its finding and recommendations respecting the application to the Secretary, acting through the Director of the National Center for Health Statistics, in such form and manner as the Secretary shall by regulation prescribe. The Secretary may not approve an application described in such subparagraph unless a peer review group has recommended the application for approval.

(C) The Secretary, acting through the Director of the National Center for Health Statistics, shall make appointments to the peer review groups required in subparagraph (A) from among persons who are not officers or employees of the United States and who possess appropriate technical and scientific qualifications, except that peer review groups regarding grants under section 306(n) may include appropriately qualified such officers and employees.

(c) The aggregate number of grants and contracts made or entered into under sections 304 and 305 for any fiscal year respecting a particular means of delivery of health services or another particular aspect of health services may not exceed twenty; and the aggregate amount of funds obligated under grants and contracts under such sections for any fiscal year respecting a particular means of delivery of health services or another particular aspect of health services may not exceed $5,000,000.

(d) No information, if an establishment or person supplying the information or described in it is identifiable, obtained in the course of activities undertaken or supported under section 304, 306, or 307 may be used for any purpose other than the purpose for which it was supplied unless such establishment or person has consented (as determined under regulations of the Secretary) to its use for such other purpose and in the case of information obtained in the course of health statistical or epidemiological activities under section 304 or 306, such information may not be published or released in other form if the particular establishment or person supplying the information or described in it is identifiable unless such establishment or person has consented (as determined under regulations of the Secretary) to its publication or release in other form.

(e)(1) Payments of any grant or under any contract under section 304, 306, or 307 may be made in advance or by way of reimbursement, and in such installments and on such conditions, as the Secretary deems necessary to carry out the purposes of such section.

(2) The amounts otherwise payable to any person under a grant or contract made under section 304, 306, or 307 shall be reduced by—

(A) amounts equal to the fair market value of any equipment or supplies furnished to such person by the Secretary for the purpose of carrying out the project with respect to which such grant or contract is made, and

(B) amounts equal to the pay, allowances, traveling expenses, and related personnel expenses attributable to the performance of services by an officer or employee of the Government in connection with such project, if such officer or employee was assigned or detailed by the Secretary to perform such services, but only if such person requested the Secretary to furnish such equipment or supplies, or such services, as the case may be.

(f) Contracts may be entered into under section 304 or 306 without regard to sections 3648 and 3709 of the Revised Statutes (31 U.S.C. 529; 41 U.S.C. 5).

(g)(1) The Secretary shall —

    (A) publish, make available, and disseminate, promptly in understandable form and on as broad a basis as practicable, the results of health services research, demonstrations, and evaluations undertaken and supported under sections 304 and 305;

    (B) make available to the public data developed in such research, demonstrations, and evaluations; and

    (C) provide indexing, abstracting, translating, publishing, and other services leading to a more effective and timely dissemination of information on health services research, demonstrations, and evaluations in health care delivery to public and private entities and individuals engaged in the improvement of health care delivery and the general public; and undertake programs to develop new or improved methods for making such information available.

(2) The Secretary shall (A) take such action as may be necessary to assure that statistics developed under sections 304 and 306 are of high quality, timely, comprehensive as well as specific, standardized, and adequately analyzed and indexed, and (B) publish, make available, and disseminate such statistics on as wide a basis as is practicable.

(h)(1) Except where the Secretary determines that unusual circumstances make a larger percentage necessary in order to effectuate the purposes of section 306, a grant or contract under any of such sections with respect to any project for construction of a facility or for acquisition of equipment may not provide for payment of more than 50 per centum of so much of the cost of the facility or equipment as the Secretary determines is reasonably attributable to research, evaluation, or demonstration purposes.

(2) Laborers and mechanics employed by contractors and subcontractors in the construction of such a facility shall be paid wages at rates not less than those prevailing on similar work in the locality, as determined by the Secretary of Labor in accordance with the Act of March 3, 1931 (40 U.S.C. 267a—267a-5, known as the Davis-Bacon Act); and the Secretary of Labor shall have with respect to any labor standards specified in this paragraph the authority and functions set forth in Reorganization Plan Numbered 14 of 1950 (5 U.S.C. Appendix) and section 2 of the Act of June 13, 1934 (40 U.S.C. 276c).

(3) Such grants and contracts shall be subject to such additional requirements as the Secretary may by regulation prescribe.

Related authorities outside the Public Health Service Act:

Public Law Number	Date	Title
95–626	11/10/78	Health Services and Centers Amendments of 1978
		Section 404 mandated the publication of a "Prevention Profile" on every three years, presenting data on health promotion and disease prevention.
101–239	12/19/89	Omnibus Budget Reconciliation Act of 1989
		Section 6507 required the development of a national system to link data from birth, infant death, and Medicaid records.
101–445	10/22/90	National Nutrition Monitoring and Related Research Act of 1990
		Mandated a coordinated, 10-year program to improve the data for monitoring nutrition status, and to improve the comparability of nutrition monitoring data collected by DHHS and USDA; established a National Nutrition Monitoring Advisory Council; and established new procedures for review and clearance of dietary guidance.
101–582	11/15/90	Year 2000 Health Objectives Planning Act of 1990
		Provides for grants to States for the development of plans to implement the Year 2000 Health Objectives within each State, including the assessment of health within the State; and mandates the development of uniform health status indicators for use by Federal, State, and local health agencies, along with model methods of collecting and reporting data.

APPENDIX E

Acronyms

The list below includes agencies, organizations, surveys, diseases, and programs.

AARP	American Association of Retired Persons
ADAMHA	Alcohol, Drug Abuse and Mental Health Administration
AHA	American Hospital Association
AHCPR	Agency for Health Care Policy and Research
AIDS	Acquired Immune Deficiency Syndrome
AMA	American Medical Association
BMAD	Part B Medicare Annual Data System
CAT	Computer-Aided Tomography
CATI	Computer Assisted Telephone Interview
CBO	Congressional Budget Office
CDC	Centers for Disease Control
CHSS	Cooperative Health Statistics System
DAWN	Drug Abuse Warning Network
DHHS	Department of Health and Human Services
DRG	Diagnosis Related Group
ESRD	End Stage Renal Disease
GAO	General Accounting Office
GNP	Gross National Product
HES	Health Examination Survey

HCFA	Health Care Financing Administration
HIV	Human Immunosuppressive Virus
HMO	Health Maintenance Organization
HRS	Health Records Survey
HSA	Health Services Area
IMCARE	Internal Medicine Center of Advance Research and Education
IOM	Institute of Medicine
JAMA	Journal of the American Medical Association
MBHSR	Medicare Beneficiary Health Status Registry
MCBS	Medicare Current Beneficiary Survey
MEDPAR	Medicare Provider Analysis and Review
MRI	Magnetic Resonance Imaging
MSA	Metropolitan Statistical Areas
NAMCS	National Ambulatory Medical Care Survey
NCHSR	National Center for Health Services Research
NCHS	National Center for Health Statistics
NCVHS	National Committee on Vital and Health Statistics
NDATUS	National Drug and Alcoholism Treatment Unit Survey
NDI	National Death Index
NGLTF	National Gay and Lesbian Task Force
NHANES	National Health and Nutrition Examination Survey
NHCS	National Health Care Survey
NHDS	National Hospital Discharge Survey
NHIS	National Health Interview Survey
NIDA	National Institute on Drug Abuse
NIAAA	National Institute on Alcohol Abuse and Alcoholism
NIH	National Institutes of Health
NIMH	National Institute of Mental Health
NMES	National Medical Expenditure Survey
NMFI	National Master Facility Inventory
NHPI	National Health Provider Inventory
NNHS	National Nursing Home Survey
OECD	Organisations for Economic Cooperation and Development
OTA	Office of Technology Assessment
PHS	Public Health Service
PPO	Preferred Provider Organization
PPS	Probability Proportional to Size
PSU	Primary Sampling Units
RAI	Resident Assessment Instrument
SAIAN	Survey of American Indians and Alaska Natives
SNF	Skilled Nursing Facilities
USPSTF	United States Preventive Services Task Force

APPENDIX F

Biographical Sketches

LINDA H. AIKEN is trustee professor of sociology and nursing at the University of Pennsylvania. At the university she directs the Center for Health Services and Policy Research and is a research associate at the Population Studies Center and senior fellow at the Leonard Davis Institute for Health Economics. Previously she was vice president of the Robert Wood Johnson Foundation, where she directed the research program. Her research interests include health care utilization surveys, the organization and finance of health care, and health manpower policy. She received bachelor's and master's degrees in nursing from the University of Florida and a Ph.D. in sociology and demography from the University of Texas, Austin.

ROBERT L. BLACK is a pediatrician in private practice in Monterey, California, as well as a clinical professor of pediatrics at Stanford University, teaching in the outpatient clinic one day a week. He is a member of the California State Maternal, Child, Adolescent Health Board. He has been active in the American Academy of Pediatrics in a number of committees and offices; currently he is chairman of the Academy's state committee on state government affairs and a member of the national committee. He is also chairman of the Academy's committee on health planning for the state of California, and senior author of its California Health Plan For Children. He has been a member of the Institute of Medicine since 1983. He has an A.B. in basic medical sciences and an M.D. from Stanford University.

JOHN W. COOMBS is director-general of the Institutions and Social Statistics Branch at Statistics Canada and former director of its Health Division. His responsibilities include the management of the national health information program in Canada. He recently has served as secretary to the National Task Force on Health Information, an examination of the current status of health information and the priority areas that it should better serve in the future, and is a member of the advisory committee to the Population Health Project of the Canadian Institute of Advanced Research. He has a B.Sc. degree in mathematics from Acadia University.

DANIEL G. HORVITZ is retired from the Research Triangle Institute, where he was executive vice president from 1983 through 1988 and vice president for statistical sciences from 1976. Most recently he was interim director of the newly created National Institute of Statistical Sciences. Previously he held academic appointments in statistics at the University of Pittsburgh, North Carolina State University, and the University of North Carolina at Chapel Hill. His major interest is in the design and methodology of large-scale social surveys. He is a fellow of the American Statistical Association; he has also served as its vice president and as chair of the survey research methods section. An elected member of the International Statistical Institute, he was program chair for its 1983 scientific meetings. He is currently chair-elect of the statistics section of the American Association for the Advancement of Science. He received a B.S. in mathematics from the University of Massachusetts and a Ph.D. in statistics from Iowa State University.

SUZANNE W. FLETCHER is editor of *Annals of Internal Medicine* and adjunct professor of the University of Pennsylvania School of Medicine. Previously she was professor of medicine and epidemiology at the University of North Carolina at Chapel Hill. Her major research interests include clinical epidemiology, health promotion and disease prevention, and screening for breast cancer. More recently she has become involved in research on the editorial process. She received a B.A. in biology from Swarthmore College, an M.D. degree from Harvard Medical School, and an M.Sc. from the Johns Hopkins School of Hygiene and Public Health.

FLOYD J. FOWLER, JR., is a senior research fellow at the Center for Survey Research, University of Massachusetts-Boston. Much of his research has dealt with sources of error in health surveys. A major focus of recent research has been measuring patient outcomes resulting from medical treatments. He received a B.A. degree from Wesleyan University and a Ph.D. in social psychology from the University of Michigan.

BIOGRAPHICAL SKETCHES

WILLIAM D. KALSBEEK is associate professor as well as director of the Survey Research Unit in the Department of Biostatistics at the University of North Carolina at Chapel Hill. He was previously a sampling statistician at the Research Triangle Institute. His recent research has dealt with cost-efficiency in survey design and the problem of sampling elusive populations. During his career he has published extensively from his experience in directing or providing significant design consultation to dozens of sample surveys. He received a B.A. in mathematics from Northwestern College in Iowa and M.P.H. and Ph.D. degrees in biostatistics from the University of Michigan.

GRAHAM KALTON became senior statistician and vice president of Westat, Inc., in January 1992. Previously he was a research scientist in the Survey Research Center, a professor of biostatistics and a professor of statistics a the University of Michigan. Prior to that he was professor of social statistics at the University of Southampton and reader in social statistics at the London School of Economics. His research interests are in survey sampling and general survey methodology. He received a B.Sc. in economics and an M.Sc. in statistics from the University of London and a Ph.D. in survey methodology from the University of Southampton. He is a fellow of the American Statistical Association and of the American Association for the Advancement of Science and the current president of the International Association of Survey Statisticians. He is a member of the Committee on National Statistics and has served as a member of its Panel to Evaluate the National Center for Education Statistics, as the chair of the Panel to Study the NSF Scientific and Technical Personnel Data System, and currently as chair of the Panel to Evaluate the Survey of Income and Program Participation.

SIDNEY KATZ is professor emeritus of gerontology and geriatrics at Columbia University and co-director of the Stroud Program on the Science of Quality of Life in Aging. His background is in medicine, epidemiology, and health services research. He investigates rehabilitation, long-term care, and the natural course of aging and chronic diseases. He has developed measures that can be used to evaluate service quality and has used these measures to develop services that enhance quality of life and quality of care. In 1987, he was guest editor of a special issue of the *Journal of Chronic Diseases* entitled the "Science of the Quality of Life." He is a member of the Institute of Medicine, serves on its Board on Health Care Services, and chaired a committee that conducted a three-year study of nursing home regulations. In the past, he has been professor at Case Western Reserve University, Michigan State University, and Brown University, where he was associate dean of medicine and director of its Gerontology

Center. Brown University established an honorary lectureship in his name, and Columbia University awarded him its Medal of Excellence in Scholarship and its Award for Excellence in Health Policy Research in Geriatrics and Gerontology. He has a B.S. in chemistry from Case Western Reserve University, an M.A. from Brown University, and an M.D. from Case Western Reserve University.

DAVID MECHANIC is director of the Institute for Health, Health Care Policy, and Aging Research at Rutgers University, a university professor, and the Rene Dubos professor of behavioral sciences. He is a member of the National Academy of Sciences and the Institute of Medicine and serves on the National Committee on Vital and Health Statistics of the Department of Health and Human Services and the Health Advisory Board of the General Accounting Office. He also serves on the Commission on Behavioral and Social Sciences and Education of the National Research Council and was vice chair of the Institute of Medicine's Committee for Pain, Disability, and Chronic Illness Behavior. Mechanic was a member of the National Institutes of Health's National Advisory Council on Aging, chair of the council's program committee, and chair of the section on social, economic and political sciences of the American Association for the Advancement of Science. He is the author of numerous books and other publications on health policy and health services research. He has a B.A. in sociology from City University of New York and M.A. and Ph.D. degrees in sociology from Stanford University.

JOSEPH P. NEWHOUSE is the John D. MacArthur professor of health policy and management at Harvard University and holds appointments on the faculties of the Kennedy School of Government, the Harvard Medical School, the Harvard School of Public Health, and the Faculty of Arts and Sciences. In addition, he directs Harvard's Division of Health Policy Research and Education and is a senior corporate fellow of the RAND Corporation, where he was the principal investigator for the RAND Health Insurance Experiment. He is the editor of the *Journal of Health Economics* and an associate editor of the *Journal of Economic Perspectives.* He is currently the chair of the Health Services Research Grants Review Committee of the Agency for Health Care Policy and Research. His recent research interests have included health care financing, medical malpractice, and costs imposed on others by cigarettes and alcohol. He is a member of the Institute of Medicine and currently serves on its council. He received both B.A. and Ph.D. degrees in economics from Harvard University.

ADRIAN M. OSTFELD is the Anna M.R. Lauder professor of epidemiology and public health at the Yale University School of Medicine and a former chairman of that department. He is a member of the Institute of Medicine. He serves on the editorial board of the *American Journal of Epidemiology*, the *Journal of Clinical Epidemiology, Psychosomatic Medicine,* and the *Journal of Behavioral Medicine*. He has been a member of the National Advisory Council on Aging of the National Institutes of Health. His primary research interests are in the epidemiology of aging and of cardiovascular disease.

EDWARD B. PERRIN (Cochair) is professor and chairman of the Department of Health Services in the School of Public Health and Community Medicine at the University of Washington. During 1991-1992 he was on sabbatical leave at Churchill College, Cambridge University. Previously he was chairman of the Department of Biostatistics at the University of Washington and the director of the Health and Population Study Center at Battelle Memorial Institute. From 1972 to 1973, he served as deputy director, and from 1973 to 1975 as director, of the National Center for Health Statistics, Department of Health, Education, and Welfare. Perrin is a member of the Institute of Medicine, serves on its Board on Health Care Services, and chairs the Committee on Clinical Evaluation of the Institute of Medicine, and is a fellow of the American Statistical Association. His areas of current research interest include mathematical modeling, large health data systems for use in decision making, and methodologies for the measurement of health care outcomes. He received a B.A. in mathematics from Middlebury College, an M.A. degree in mathematical statistics from Columbia University, and a Ph.D. in statistics from Stanford University.

WILLIAM C. RICHARDSON (Cochair) is president of the Johns Hopkins University. Previously he was executive vice president and provost of Pennsylvania State University and prior to that graduate dean and vice provost for research at the University of Washington, Seattle. He joined the University of Washington as a faculty member in the School of Public Health and Community Medicine and went on to become chairman of the Department of Health Services and associate dean of the School of Public Health and professor of health services. His areas of research have included use of health services by various enrolled populations and comparisons of access, quality, and costs under differing managed care arrangements. He is a member of the Institute of Medicine and a fellow of the American Public Health Association. Richardson has a B.A. from Trinity College (Hartford, Connecticut), and M.B.A. and Ph.D. degrees from the University of Chicago Graduate School of Business.

GOOLOO S. WUNDERLICH (study director) is a member of the staff of the Committee on National Statistics. She has over 30 years of experience in health and population statistics and research in the U.S. Public Health Service, the Presidential Advisory Commission on Rural Poverty, the Bureau of the Census, and as a consultant. She is a former director of the Division of Data Policy, Office of the Assistant Secretary for Health in the Department of Health and Human Services, serving for many years as the focus for data policy analysis, development, planning, and coordination of health information systems and statistical activities; she also directed the review and approval of statistical, research, and regulatory data collection activities throughout the U.S. Public Health Service. Her professional interests and experience have focused on the conduct and analysis of national health surveys, analysis and policy formulation relating to population research, family planning and health issues. She received B.A., M.A., and Ph.D. degrees from the University of Bombay, India; she completed two years of postdoctoral studies in sociology, statistics, and demography at the universities of Minnesota and Chicago.

Sources and References

Aaron, H.J.
    1991a Looking Backward: 2001-1991. The History of the Health Care Financing and Reform Act of 1988. *The Brookings Review* 40-45 (Summer).
    1991b *Serious and Unstable Condition: Financing Americans' Health Care.* Washington, DC: The Brookings Institution.

Aaron, H.J., and W.B. Schwartz
    1984 *The Painful Prescription: Rationing Hospital Care.* Washington, DC: The Brookings Institution.
    1990 Rationing Health Care: The Choice Before Us. *Science* 247: 418-422.

Aiken, L.H., and C.F. Mullinex
    1987 The Nursing Shortage: Myth or Reality? *New England Journal of Medicine* 317:641-646.

Aiken, L.H., M.D. Mezey, J.E. Lynaugh, and C.R. Buck, Jr.
    1985 Teaching Nursing Homes: Prospects for Improving Long-term Care. *Journal of the American Geriatrics Society* 33 (3 March):196-201.

Altman, S.H., and R. Blendon
    1979 *Medical Technology: The Culprit Behind Health Care Costs?* DHEW Publication No. (PHS) 79-3216. Rockville, MD: U.S. Public Health Service.

American Association of Retired Persons (AARP)
    1991a *Medicare: Meeting the Health Care Needs of the Elderly.* Issue Brief No. 7, July. Washington, DC: American Association of Retired Persons.
    1991b *Physician Payment Reform Under Medicare.* Issue Brief No. 8, August. Washington, DC: American Association of Retired Persons.

American Hospital Association (AHA)
  1988   *Annual Survey of Hospitals.* Chicago: AHA.
American Medical Association (AMA)
  1989   Annual Education Issue. *Journal of the American Medical Association.*
  1990a *Attributes to Guide the Development of Practice Parameters.* Chicago: AMA.
  1990b *Directory of Practice Parameters.* Chicago: AMA.
  1991   Caring for the Uninsured and Underinsured. Special Issue. *Journal of the American Medical Association* 265(19):2491-2567.
Anderson, G.F., C.J. Schramm, C.R. Rapoza, et al.
  1985   Investor-Owned Chains and Teaching Hospitals: The Implications of Acquisition. *The New England Journal of Medicine* 313:201-204.
Andrulis, D.P., V.S. Beers, and L.S. Gage
  1989   The 1987 U.S. Hospital AIDS Survey. *Journal of the American Medical Association* 262(6):784-794.
Audet, A., S. Greenbert, and M. Field
  1990   Medical Practice Guidelines: Current Activities and Future Directions. *Annals of Internal Medicine* 113:709-714.
Banta, H.D., C.J. Behney, and J.S. Willems
  1981   *Toward Rational Technology in Medicine.* Springer Series on Health Care and Society. New York: Springer Publishing Company.
Barry, M.J., A.G. Mulley, F.J. Fowler, et al.
  1988   Watchful Waiting vs. Immediate Transurethral Resection for Symptomatic Prostatism: The Importance of Patients' Preferences. *Journal of the American Medical Association* 259:3010-3017.
Batalden, P.B., and E.D. Buchanan
  1989   Industrial Models of Quality Improvement. Pp. 133-159 in N. Goldfield and D.B. Nash, eds., *Providing Quality Care: The Challenge to Clinicians.* Philadelphia: American College of Physicians.
Berwick, D.M.
  1989   Sounding Board: Continuous Improvement as an Ideal in Health Care. *New England Journal of Medicine* 320:53-56.
Berwick, D.M., A.B. Godfrey, and J. Roessner
  1990   *Curing Health Care. New Strategies for Quality Improvement.* San Francisco: Jossey-Bass Publishers.
Blendon, R.J., and J.N. Edwards
  1991   Caring for the Uninsured: Choices for Reform. *Journal of the American Medical Association* 265:2563-2565.
Bloom, B.
  1990   Health Insurance and Medical Care. Health of Our Nation's Children, United States, 1988. Advance Data from Vital and Health Statistics. No. 188. Hyattsville, MD: National Center for Health Statistics, October 1.
Boruch, R., and R. Pearson
  1988   Assessing the Quality of Longitudinal Surveys. *Evaluation Review* 12(1):3-58.

Brickner, P.W., L.K. Scharer, B.A. Conanan, M. Savarese, and B.C. Scanlan
- 1990 *Under the Safety Net: The Health and Social Welfare of the Homeless in the United States.* A United Hospital Fund Book. New York: W.W. Norton & Company.

Brook, R.H.
- 1989 Practice Guidelines and Practicing Medicine: Are They Compatible? *Journal of the American Medical Association* 262:3027-3030.
- 1990 Practice Guidelines (In Reply). *Journal of the American Medical Association* 263:3022.
- 1991 Health, Health Insurance, and the Uninsured. *Journal of the American Medical Association* 265:2998-3002.

Brook, R.H., A.D. Avery, S. Greenfield, et al.
- 1976 *Quality of Medical Care Assessment Using Outcomes Measures. An Overview of the Method.* R-2021/1-HEW. Santa Monica, CA: The RAND Corporation.

Brook, R.H., and K.N. Lohr
- 1985 Efficacy, Effectiveness, Variations, and Quality: Boundary Crossing Research. *Medical Care* 23:710-722.
- 1986 Will We Need to Ration Effective Health Care? *Issues in Science and Technology* 3(1): 68-77.

Brown, Lawrence D.
- 1988 *Health Policy in the United States: Issues and Options.* Occasional Paper 4, Ford Foundation Project on Social Welfare and the American Future. New York: Ford Foundation.
- 1991 The National Politics of Oregon's Rationing Debate. *Health Affairs* 10(2):28-51.

Bureau of the Census
- 1960 *Historical Statistics of the United States, Colonial Times to 1957.* Washington, DC: U.S. Department of Commerce.

Burns, L.A., and D.M. Mancino
- 1987 *Joint Ventures Between Hospitals and Physicians: A Competitive Strategy for the Healthcare Marketplace.* Homewood, IL: Dow Jones-Irwin.

Butler, S.M.
- 1991 A Tax Reform Strategy to Deal with the Uninsured. *Journal of the American Medical Association* 265:2541-2544.

Callahan, D.
- 1987 *Setting Limits: Medical Goals in an Aging Society.* New York: Simon and Schuster.
- 1990 *What Kind of Life: The Limits of Medical Progress.* New York: Simon and Schuster.
- 1991 Commentary: Ethics and Priority Setting in Oregon. *Health Affairs* 10(2):78-87.

Cantor, J.C., N.L. Barrand, R.A. Desonia, A.B. Cohen, and J.C. Merrill.
- 1991 Business Leaders' Views on American Health Care. *Health Affairs* DataWatch 11(1):98-105.

Chassin, M.R.
- 1988 Standards of Care in Medicine. *Inquiry* 25:437-450.

Citro, C.F., and E.A. Hanushek, eds.
- 1991 *Improving Information for Social Policy Decisions. The Uses of Microsimulation Modeling.* Volume I: Review and Recommendations. Panel to Evaluate Microsimulation Models for Social Welfare Programs, Committee on National Statistics. Washington, DC: National Academy Press.

Cochran, William G.
- 1976 The Role of Statistics in National Health Policy Decisions. *American Journal of Epidemiology* 104(4):370-379.

Commission on Life Sciences, NRC
- 1991 *Mapping and Sequencing the Human Genome.* National Research Council. Washington, DC: National Academy Press.

Congressional Budget Office
- 1991a *Rising Health Care Costs: Causes, Implications, and Strategies.* Washington, DC: U.S. Government Printing Office.
- 1991b *Restructuring Health Insurance for Medicare Enrollees.* Washington, DC: U.S. Government Printing Office.

Cox, B., and S.B. Cohen
- 1985 *Methodological Issues for Health Care Surveys.* New York: Marcek Dekker.

Cox, Brenda G., R.E. Folsom, and T.G. Virag
- 1987 *Design Alternatives for Integrating the National Medical Expenditures Survey With the National Health Interview Survey.* DHHS Publication No. (PHS) 87-1375. Hyattsville, MD: National Center for Health Statistics.

Donabedian, A.
- 1966 Evaluating the Quality of Medical Care. *Milbank Memorial Fund Quarterly* 44:166-203 (July, Part 2).
- 1980 *Explorations in Quality Assessment and Monitoring.* Volume I. Ann Arbor, MI: Health Administration Press.
- 1982 *Explorations in Quality Assessment and Monitoring.* Volume II. Ann Arbor, MI: Health Administration Press.
- 1985 *Explorations in Quality Assessment and Monitoring.* Volume III. Ann Arbor, MI: Health Administration Press.

Duncan, G., and G. Kalton
- 1987 Issues of Design and Analysis of Survey Across Time. *International Statistical Review* 55(1):97-117.

Duncan, J.W., and W.C. Shelton
- 1978 *Revolution in United States Government Statistics, 1926-1976.* Office of Federal Statistical Policy and Standards, October. Washington, DC: U.S. Department of Commerce.

Eddy, D.M., ed.
- 1991 *Common Screening Tests.* Philadelphia: American College of Physicians.
- Forthcoming *A Manual for Assessing Health Practices and Designing Practice Policies.* Philadelphia: American College of Physicians (in collaboration with the Council of Medical Specialty Societies).

SOURCES AND REFERENCES

Ellwood, P.M.
1988 The Shattuck Lecture: Outcomes Management. A Technology of Patient Experience. *New England Journal of Medicine* 318:1549-1566.

Erickson, P., E.A. Kendall, J.P. Anderson, and R.M. Kaplan
1989 Using Composite Health Status Measures to Assess the Nation's Health. *Medical Care* 27(3): S66-S76 (March Supplement).

Ermann, D., and J. Gabel
1985 The Changing Face of American Health Care: Multihospital Systems, Emergency Centers and Surgery Centers. *Medical Care* 23:401-420.

Etzioni, A.
1991 Health Care Rationing: A Critical Evaluation. *Health Affairs* 10(2): 88-95.

Fletcher, R., and S. Fletcher
1990 Clinical Practice Guidelines. *Annals of Internal Medicine* 113:645-646.

Flexner, A.
1910 *Medical Education in the United States and Canada: A Report to the Carnegie Foundation for the Advancement of Teaching.* Bulletin No. 4. New York: Carnegie Foundation.

Fowler, F.J., J.E. Wennberg, R.P. Timothy, et al.
1988 Symptom Status and Quality of Life Following Prostatectomy. *Journal of the American Medical Association* 259:2018-3022.

Fox, D.M., and H.M. Leichter
1991 Rationing Care in Oregon: The New Accountability. *Health Affairs* 10(2):7-27.

Frank, E., R.F. Prien, R.B. Jarrett, M.B. Keller, D.J. Kupfer, P.W. Lavori, A.J. Rush, and M.M. Weissman
1991 Conceptualization and Rationale for Consensus Definitions of Terms in Major Depressive Disorder: Remission, Recovery, Relapse, and Recurrence. *Archives of General Psychiatry* 48(9 September):851-855.

Frenzen, P.D.
1991 The Increasing Supply of Physicians in US Urban and Rural Areas, 1975 to 1988. *American Journal of Public Health* 81:1141-1147.

Gelijns, A.C.
1991 *Innovation in Clinical Practice. The Dynamics of Medical Technology Development.* Washington, DC: National Academy Press.

General Accounting Office
1991 *Practice Guidelines: The Experience of Medical Specialty Societies.* GAO/PEMD-91-11. Washington, DC: General Accounting Office.

Gilford, Dorothy M., ed.
1988 *The Aging Population in the Twenty-First Century: Statistics for Health Policy.* Panel on Statistics for an Aging Population, Committee on National Statistics, Commission on Behavioral and Social Sciences and Education, National Research Council. Washington, DC: National Academy Press.

Ginzberg, E.
1984 The Monetarization of Medical Care. *The New England Journal of Medicine* 310:1162-1166.

Goldfield, N., and D.B. Nash, eds.
1989 *Providing Quality Care: The Challenge to Clinicians.* Philadelphia: American College of Physicians.

Grannemann, T.W.
1991 Priority Setting: A Sensible Approach to Medicaid Policy? *Inquiry* 38:300-305.

Haglund, K.
1991 Health-Care Reform Plans: Is Universal, Affordable Access to Care Really Coming? *The Journal of NIH Research* 3 (July):35-37.

Harper, T., M. Berlin, R. DiGaetano, D. Walsh, and J. Ingels
1991 *National Medical Expenditure Survey, Household Survey, Final Methodology Report.* Rockville, MD: Westat, Inc.

Harris-Wehling, J.
1990 Oral and Written Testimony from the Public Hearings. Pp. 7-34 in K.N. Lohr, ed., *Medicare: A Strategy for Quality Assurance. Volume II. Sources and Methods.* Institute of Medicine. Washington, DC: National Academy Press.

Health Affairs
1988 Special Issue. The Pursuit of Quality. *Health Affairs* 7(1):3-150.
1991 Special Issue. Pursuit of Health Systems Reform. *Health Affairs* 10(3):4-268.

Heckman, J.J., and B. Singer
1985 *Longitudinal Analysis of Labor Market Data.* New York: Cambridge University Press.

Hellinger, F.J.
1990 Updated Forecasts of the Costs of Medical Care for Persons with AIDS, 1989-1993. *Public Health Reports* 105(1):1-12.

Himmelstein, D.U., and S. Woolhandler
1989 A National Health Program for the United States: A Physician's Proposal. *New England Journal of Medicine* 320:102-108.

Hornbrook, M.C., A.V. Hurtado, and R.E. Johnson
1985 Health Care Episodes: Definition, Measurement and Use. *Medical Care Review* 42(2):163-218.

Inquiry
1988 Special Issue. The Challenge of Quality. *Inquiry* 25:3-194.

Institute of Medicine
1985 *Assessing Medical Technologies.* Committee for Evaluating Medical Technologies in Clinical Use. Washington, DC: National Academy Press.
1988 *Homelessness, Health, and Human Needs.* Washington, DC: National Academy Press.
1989a *Controlling Costs and Changing Patient Care? The Role of Utilization Management.* B.H. Gray and M.J. Field, eds. Washington, DC: National Academy Press.
1989b *Medical Professional Liability and the Delivery of Obstetrical Care.* Washington, DC: National Academy Press.
1989c *Allied Health Services: Avoiding Crises.* Washington, DC: National Academy Press.

1990a Breast Cancer: Setting Priorities for Effectiveness Research. K.N. Lohr, ed. Washington, DC: National Academy Press.
1990b Clinical Practice Guidelines: Directions for a New Program. M.J. Field and K.N. Lohr, eds. Washington, DC: National Academy Press.
1990c Medicare: A Strategy for Quality Assurance. Volume I. K.N. Lohr, ed. Washington, DC: National Academy Press.
1990d Effectiveness and Outcomes in Health Care. Proceedings of a Conference. Heithoff, K.A. and K.N. Lohr, eds. Washington, DC: National Academy Press.
1991a Kidney Failure and the Federal Government. R.A. Rettig and N.G. Levinsky, eds. Washington, DC: National Academy Press.
1991b The Artificial Heart: Prototypes, Policies, and Patients. J.R. Hogness and M. VanAntwerp, eds. Washington, DC: National Academy Press.
1991c Biomedical Politics. K.E. Hanna, ed. Washington, DC: National Academy Press.
1991d Disability in America: Toward a National Agenda for Prevention. A.M. Pope and A.R. Tarlov, eds. Washington, DC: National Academy Press.
1990-1992 Medical Innovation at the Crossroads. Volumes I, II, and III, A.C. Gelijns ed. Volume II. The Changing Economics of Medical Technology, A.C. Gelijns and E.A. Halm, eds. Volume III. Health Care in Tighter Times—Roles for Patients, Providers, Innovators, A.C. Gelijns, ed. Washington, DC: National Academy Press.
1992 Guidelines for Clinical Practice: From Development to Use. M.J. Field and K.N. Lohr, eds. Washington, DC: National Academy Press.

Internal Medicine Center of Advance Research and Education (IMCARE)
1990 Medical Practice Guidelines Workshop: Issues for Internal Medicine. Washington, DC: IMCARE.

Jensen, G.A., M.A. Morrissey, and J.A. Marcus
1987 Cost Sharing and the Changing Pattern of Employer-Sponsored Health Insurance. The Milbank Quarterly 65 (Fall):521-550.

Johnson, C.M., L. Miranda, A. Sherman, and J.C. Weill
1991 Child Poverty in America. Washington, DC: Children's Defense Fund.

Kahn, K.L., L.V. Rubenstein, D. Draper, J. Kosecoff, W.H. Rogers, E.B. Keeler, and R.H. Brook
1990a Effects of the DRG-based Prospective Payment System on Quality of Care for Hospitalized Medicare Patients: An Introduction to the Series. Journal of the American Medical Association 264:1953-1955.

Kahn, K.L., E.B. Keeler, M.J. Sherwood, W.H. Rogers, D. Draper, S.S. Bentow, E.J. Reinisch, L.V. Rubenstein, J. Kosecoff, and R.H. Brook
1990b Comparing Outcomes of Care Before and After Implementation of the DRG-based Prospective Payment System. Journal of the American Medical Association 264:1984-1988.

Kalton, G., and D.W. Anderson
1986 Sampling Rare Populations. The Journal of the Royal Statistical Society Series A (General) 149 (Part 1):65-82.

Kalton, G., D. Kasprzyk, and D.B. McMillen
1989 Nonsampling Errors in Panel Surveys. In D. Kasprzyk et al., eds., Panel Surveys. New York: John Wiley and Sons.

Kasprzyk, D., and C. Jacobs
    1991   Federal Longitudinal Surveys. Pp. 303-406 in *Seminar on Quality of Federal Data*. Statistical Policy Working Paper, No. 20. National Technical Information Service, PB91-142414.

Kasprzyk, D., G. Duncan, G. Kalton, and M.P. Singh, eds.
    1989   *Panel Surveys*. New York: J.W. Wiley and Sons, Inc.

Kass, N.E., R.R. Faden, R. Fox, and J. Dudley
    1991   Loss of Private Health Insurance Among Homosexual Men with AIDS. *Inquiry* 28: 249-254.

Katz, S., guest ed.
    1987   The Portugal Conference: Measuring Quality of Life and Functional Status in Clinical and Epidemiologic Research. Proceedings. *Journal of Chronic Diseases* 40(6):459-650.

Keeler, E.B.
    1991   Uses of Episodes of Care in Effectiveness Research. Discussion paper presented at Medical Effectiveness Research Data Methods Conference, Minneapolis, September 13.

Keeler, E.B., W.G. Manning, and K.B. Wells
    1988   The Demand for Episodes of Mental Health Services. *Journal of Health Economics* (7):369-392.

Keeler, E.B., and J.E. Rolph
    1988   The Demand for Episodes of Treatment in the Health Insurance Experiment. *Journal of Health Economics* (7):337-367.

Kleinman, Joel C., and D. Makuc
    1983   Travel for Ambulatory Medical Care. *Medical Care* 21(5):543-557.

Laumann, E., and D. Knoke
    1987   *The Organizational State: Social Choice in National Policy Domains*. Madison: University of Wisconsin Press.

Lazenby, H.C., and S.W. Letsch
    1990   National Health Expenditures, 1989. *Health Care Financing Review* 12(2):2-26.

Leape, L.
    1990   Practice Guidelines and Standards: An Overview. *QRB (Quality Review Bulletin)* 16:42-49.

Levinsky, N.G., and R.A. Rettig
    1991   Special Report. The Medicare End-Stage Renal Disease Program. A Report from the Institute of Medicine. *New England Journal of Medicine* 324:1143-1148.

Levit, K.R., H.C. Lazenby, S.W. Letsch, and C.A. Cowan.
    1991   National Health Care Spending, 1989. *Health Affairs* DataWatch 10(1):117-130.

Lohr, K.N.
    1988   Outcome Measurement: Concepts and Questions. *Inquiry* 25(1):37-50.

Lohr, K.N., guest ed.
    1989   Advances in Health Status Assessment. Proceedings of a Conference. *Medical Care* 27(3):SI-S294 (March Supplement).

Lohr, K.N., and J. Durch
  1991 Summary of a Planning Meeting: Database Development for Clinical Evaluation. Unpublished Summary of IOM Program Initiation Fund Meeting. Division of Health Care Services, Institute of Medicine, August.

Lohr, K.N., and J.E. Ware, Jr., guest eds.
  1987 Proceedings of the Advances in Health Assessment Conference. *Journal of Chronic Diseases* 40:SI-S193 (First Supplement).

Lohr, K.N., K.D. Yordy, and S.O. Thier
  1988 Current Issues in Quality of Care. *Health Affairs* 7(1): 5-18.

Luft, Harold S.
  1981 *Health Maintenance Organizations: Dimensions of Performance.* New York: John Wiley & Sons, Inc.
  1991 Commentary. Translating the U.S. HMO Experience to Other Health Systems. *Health Affairs* 10(3):172-186.

Luft, Harold S., S.S. Hunt, and S.C. Maerki
  1987 The Volume-Outcome Relationship: Practice Makes Perfect or Selective Referral Patterns? *Health Services Research* 24:157-188.

Makuc, Diane M., B. Haglund, D.D. Ingram, J.C. Kleinman, and J.J. Feldman
  1990 Use of Cluster Analysis to Identify Health Care Service Areas. National Center or Health Statistics. *1990 Proceedings of the Social Statistics Section of the American Statistical Association*, pp. 260-265.

Marder, W.D., D.W. Emmons, P.R. Kletke, and R.J. Willke
  1988 Physician Employment Patterns: Challenging Conventional Wisdom. *Health Affairs* (Winter).

Marmor, T.R., and J.L. Mashaw
  1990 Canada's Health Insurance and Ours: The Real Lessons, the Real Choices. *The American Prospect* 1(3):18-29.

Mechanic, D.
  1987 Health Issues in an Aging Society: The Research Agenda. *Proceedings of the 1987 Public Health Conference on Records and Statistics*, Department of Health and Human Services, Pub. No. 88-1214, pp. 17-20.

Meehan, P.J., L.E. Saltzman, R.W. Sattin
  1991 Suicides Among Older United States Residents: Epidemiologic Characteristics and Trends. *American Journal of Public Health* 81: 1198-1200.

Mosteller, F., and J. Falotico-Taylor, eds.
  1989 *Quality of Life and Technology Assessment.* Monograph of the Council on Health Care Technology. Washington, DC: National Academy Press.

Nathan, Gad
  1976 An Empirical Study of Response and Sampling Errors for Multiplicity Estimates with Different Counting Rules. *Journal of the American Statistical Association* 71(356) Applications Section: 808-815.

National Center for Health Services Research (NCHSR)
  1988 Patient Outcomes Assessment Research Program: Extramural Assessment Teams. *NCHSR Program Note.* Rockville, MD: U.S. Department of Health and Human Services.

National Center for Health Statistics
- 1963 Origin, Program, and Operation of the U.S. National Health Survey. Vital and Health Statistics, Series 1, Number 1, U.S. Department of Health, Education, and Welfare, Public Health Service, August.
- 1964 Health Survey Procedure: Concepts, Questionnaire Development, and Definitions in the Health Interview Survey. Vital and Health Statistics, Series 1, Number 2, U.S. Department of Health, Education, and Welfare, Public Health Service, May.
- 1965 Origin, Program, and Operation of the U.S. National Health Survey. Vital and Health Statistics, Series 1, Number 1, U.S. Department of Health, Education, and Welfare, Public Health Service.
- 1966 *History of the United States National Committee on Vital and Health Statistics, 1949-1964.* Vital and Health Statistics, Series 4, Number 5, U.S. Department of Health, Education, and Welfare, Public Health Service.
- 1973 Plan and Initial Program of the Health Examination Survey, Vital and Health Statistics, Series 1, Number 4, U.S. Department of Health, Education, and Welfare, Public Health Service, Health Resources Administration.
- 1975 The Analytical Potential of NCHS Data for Health Care Systems: A Report of the United States National Committee on Vital and Health Statistics. Vital and Health Statistics, Series 4, Number 17, U.S. Department of Health, Education, and Welfare, Public Health Service.
- 1981 Discharge from Nursing Homes. Series 13, Number 54. DHEW Publication No. (PHS) 81-1715. Hyattsville, MD.
- 1989b *Health United States 1988.* DHHS Publication No. (PHS) 89-1232. Hyattsville, MD: U.S Public Health Service.
- 1989c *Health United States 1989.* DHHS Publication No. (PHS) 90-1232. Hyattsville, MD: U.S. Public Health Service.
- 1991a *Health United States 1990.* DHHS Publication No. (PHS) 91-1232. Hyattsville, MD: U.S. Public Health Service.
- 1991b Current Legislative Authorities of the National Center for Health Statistics. Enacted as of November 1990. U.S. Department of Health and Human Services, Public Health Service, Hyattsville, MD.
- 1991c Health Service Areas for the United States. Vital and Health Statistics, Series 2, Number 112, U.S. Department of Health and Human Services, Public Health Service, November.

National Gay and Lesbian Task Force Policy Institute
- 1990-1991 Current Recognition of Non-Traditional and Diverse Families. Unpublished policy paper distributed by the NGLTF, Washington, DC.

Newhouse, J.P., A.P. Williams, B.W. Bennett, and W.B. Schwartz
- 1982 Where Have All the Doctors Gone? *Journal of the American Medical Association* 247: 2392-2396.

Nutter, D.
- 1984 Access to care and the evolution of corporate, for-profit medicine. *The New England Journal of Medicine* 311: 917-919.

Office of Management and Budget
   1986   Federal Longitudinal Surveys. Statistical Policy Working Paper, No. 13, National Technical Information Service, PB86-139730.

Office of National Cost Estimates
   1990   National Health Expenditures, 1988. *Health Care Financing Review* 11(4):1-43.

Office of National Health Statistics
   1991   Data tables from *Office of the Actuary, Health Care Financing Administration*. July and August 1991. Washington, DC: U.S. Department of Health and Human Services.

Office of Technology Assessment (OTA)
   1982   *Strategies for Medical Technology Assessment*. September. Washington, DC: OTA.
   1986   *Nurse Practitioners, Physician Assistants, and Certified Nurse-Midwives; A Policy Analysis*. OTA-HCS-37. December. Washington, DC: OTA.
   1988   *The Quality of Medical Care. Information for Consumers*. OTA-H-386. June. Washington, DC: OTA.

Palmer, R.H., A. Donabedian, and G.J. Povar
   1991   *Striving for Quality in Health Care. An Inquiry into Policy and Practice*. Ann Arbor, MI: Health Administration Press.

Patrick, D.L., and M. Bergner
   1990   Measurement of Health Status in the 1990s. *Annual Review of Public Health* 11:165-183.

Patrick, D.L., and P. Erickson
   1988   What Constitutes Quality of Life? Concepts and Definitions. *Quality of Life and Cardiovascular Care* 4:103-127.

Pearson, R.
   1989   The Advantages and Disadvantages of Longitudinal Surveys. *Research in the Sociology of Education and Socialization* (8):177-199.

Peet, J.
   1991   Health Care. *The Economist* July 6:3-22.

Prien, R.F., L.L. Carpenter, and D.J. Kupfer
   1991   The Definition and Operational Criteria for Treatment Outcome of Major Depressive Disorder: A Review of the Current Research Literature. *Archives of General Psychiatry* 48(9 September):796-800.

Reinhardt, U.E.
   1991   Breaking American Health Policy Gridlock. *Health Affairs* 10(2):96-103.

Relman A.S.
   1980   The New Medical Industrial Complex. *The New England Journal of Medicine* 303:963-970.

Rice, D.P.
   1986   The Medical Care System: Past Trends and Future Projections. *The New York Medical Quarterly* 6(1):39-70.
   1989   Demographics and Health of the Elderly: Past Trends and Projections. Unpublished paper prepared for the Prospective Payment Advisory Assessment Commission.

1989 Demographic Realities and Projections of An Aging Population. Pp. 15-44 in S. Andreopoulos and J.R. Hogness, eds., *Health Care for An Aging Society*. New York: Churchill Livingstone.

Rice, D.P., and J.J. Feldman
1983 Living Longer in the United States: Demographic Changes and Health Needs of the Elderly. *Milbank Memorial Fund Quarterly* 61:362-396.

Rice, D.P., and M.P. LaPlante
1988 Chronic Illness, Disability, and Increasing Longevity. Pp. 9-55 in S. Sullivan and M.E. Lewin, eds., *The Economics and Ethics of Long-Term Care and Disability*. Washington, DC: American Enterprise Institute for Public Policy Research.

Ries, P.
1991 Characteristics of Persons With and Without Health Care Coverage: United States, 1989. *Advance Data from Vital and Health Statistics*. No. 201., June 18. Hyattsville, MD: National Center for Health Statistics.

Roper, W.L., W.L. Winkenwerder, G.M. Hackbarth, and H. Krakauer
1988 Effectiveness in Health Care: An Initiative to Evaluate and Improve Medical Practice. *New England Journal of Medicine* 319:1197-1202.

Rosenberg, M.L., J.C. Smith, L.E. Davidson, and J.M. Conn
1987 The Emergence of Youth Suicide: An Epidemiologic Analysis and Public Health Perspective. *Annual Review of Public Health* 8: 417-440.

Rossiter, L.F.
1984 Prospects for Medical Group Practice Under Competition. *Medical Care* 22:84-92.

Ruggles, P.
1991 Longitudinal Analysis of Federal Survey Data. Pp. 425-437 in *Seminar on Quality of Federal Data*. Statistical Policy Working Paper, No. 20. National Technical Information Service, PB91-142414.

Schieber, G.J., and J.P. Poullier
1988 International Health Spending and Utilization Trends. *Health Affairs* 7(3):105-112.
1989 Overview of International Comparisons of Health Care Expenditures. *Health Care Financing Review* 10: Annual Supplement.

Schieber, G.J., J.P. Poullier, and L.M. Greenwald
1991 Health Care Systems in Twenty-Four Countries. *Health Affairs* 10(3): 22-38.

Shaughnessy, P.W., A.M. Kramer, and D.F. Hittle
1990 The Teaching Nursing Home Experiment: Its Effects and Implications. Study Paper 6, Center for Health Services Research, University of Colorado, March.

Shimizu, I., and E. Cole
1990 A Comparison of Relative Standard Errors Between 2 and 3-Stage Sample Designs for NHDS. Unpublished paper, October 25. Hyattsville, MD: National Center for Health Statistics.

Short, P.F.
- 1990 Estimates of the Uninsured Population, Calendar Year 1987. *National Medical Expenditures Survey Data Summary 2.* DHHS Publication No. (PHS) 90-3469. Rockville, MD: Agency for Health Care Policy and Research, U.S. Public Health Service, September.

Sipes-Metzler, P.R.
- 1991 Oregon's Challenge to Achieve Health Care Equity. Paper prepared for a Conference on Designing a Fair and Reasonable Basic Benefit Plan Using Clinical Guidelines Sponsored by the California Public Employees Retirement System, Sacramento, CA, April 24-26, 1991.

Sirken, Monroe G.
- 1970 Household Surveys with Multiplicity. *Journal of the American Statistical Association* 65(329):257-266.
- 1972a Stratified Sample Surveys with Multiplicity. *Journal of the American Statistical Association* 67(337): 224-227.
- 1972b Variance Components of Multiplicity Estimators. *Biometrics* 28: 869-873.

Somers, H.M., and A.R. Somers
- 1961 *Doctors, Patients, and Health Insurance. The Organization and Financing of Medical Care.* Washington, DC: The Brookings Institution.

Special Committee on Aging, U.S. Congress, Senate
- 1987-1988 *Aging America: Trends and Projections, 1987-1988 Edition.* Prepared by the U.S. Senate Special Committee on Aging in conjunction with the American Association of Retired Persons, the Federal Council on the Aging, and the Administration on Aging. Washington, DC: U.S. Department of Health and Human Services.

Starfield, B.
- 1991 Primary Care and Health: A Cross-National Comparison. *Journal of the American Medical Association* 266:2268-2271.

Starfield, B., J. Weiner, L. Mumford, and D. Steinwachs
- 1991 Ambulatory Care Groups: A Categorization of Diagnoses for Research and Management. *Health Services Research* 26(1):53-74.

Starr, Paul
- 1982 *The Social Transformation of American Medicine.* New York: Basic Books, Inc., Publishers.

Steinwachs, Donald M.
- 1991 Episode of Care Framework: Utility for Medical Effectiveness Research. Paper presented the Medical Effectiveness Research Data Methods Conference, Minneapolis, MN, September 13, 1991. Steinwachs, Director and Professor, Health Services Research and Development Center, John Hopkins School of Hygiene and Public Health.

Stevens, Rosemary
- 1989 *In Sickness and In Wealth.* New York: Basic Books, Inc.

Stoto, M.A.
- 1992 Public Health Assessment in the 1990s. *Annual Review of Public Health* 11.

Sudman, S., and G. Kalton
- 1986 New Developments in the Sampling of Special Populations. *Annual Review of Sociology* 12:401-429.

Sudman, S., M.G. Sirken, and C.D. Cowan
- 1988 Sampling Rare and Elusive Populations. *Science* 240:991-995.

Sullivan, C.B., and T. Rice
- 1991 The Health Insurance Picture in 1990. *Health Affairs* DataWatch 10(2):104-115.

Tarlov, A.R.
- 1983 Shattuck Lecture—The Increasing Supply of Physicians, the Changing Structure of the Health Services System, and the Future Practice of Medicine. *The New England Journal of Medicine* 308:1235-1244.

Tarlov, A.R., J.E. Ware, Jr., S. Greenfield, E.C. Nelson, E. Perrin, and M. Zubkoff
- 1989 The Medical Outcomes Study. An Application of Methods for Monitoring the Results of Medical Care. *The Journal of the American Medical Association* 262(7):925-930.

Thomas, L.
- 1972 *Aspects of Biomedical Science Policy.* IOM Occasional Paper, p. 25. Washington, DC: Institute of Medicine.
- 1977 On the Science and Technology of Medicine. In J.H. Knowles, ed., *Doing Better and Feeling Worse: Health in the United States.* New York: W. W. Norton & Company.

Torrens, P.R.
- 1978 *The American Health Care System: Issues and Problems.* St. Louis, MO: Mosby.

U.S. Bipartisan Commission on Comprehensive Health Care (Pepper Commission)
- 1990 *A Call for Action.* Final Report of the Commission. Senate Print 101-114. September. Washington, DC: U.S. Government Printing Office.

U.S. Department of Health and Human Services
- 1986 HHS Data Inventory. Fiscal Year 1985. March.
- 1987a National Institute on Drug Abuse (NIDA). *Final Report: National Drug & Alcoholism Treatment Unit Survey (NDATUS), 1987.* NIDA, Division of Epidemiology and Prevention Research and National Institute of Alcohol Abuse and Alcoholism, Division of Biometry and Epidemiology, Rockville, MD.
- 1987b National Institute of Mental Health (NIMH) (1987). *The Inventory of Mental Health Organizations.* NIMH, Survey and Reports Branch, Rockville, MD.
- 1988b *Secretary's Commission on Nursing. Final Report.* Volume I. December. Washington, DC: U.S. Department of Health and Human Services.
- 1988c *Secretary's Commission on Nursing. Support Studies and Background Information.* Volume II. December. Washington, DC: U.S. Department of Health and Human Services.
- 1988d *Secretary's Commission on Nursing. Interim Report.* Volume III. December. Washington, DC: U.S. Department of Health and Human Services.

SOURCES AND REFERENCES

1989a HHS Data Inventory. Fiscal Year 1988. April.
1990 *Mental Health, United States, 1990*. Ronald W. Manderscheid and Mary Ann Sonnenschein, eds. National Institute of Mental Health, Public Health Service, Alcohol, Drug Abuse, and Mental Health Administration.
1991a *Healthy People 2000. National Health Promotion and Disease Prevention Objectives*. DHHS Publication No. (PHS) 91-50212. Washington, DC: Office of the Assistant Secretary for Health.
1991b The HIV/AIDS Epidemic: The First 10 Years. Morbidity and Mortality Weekly Report, June 7, 1991, Vol. 40, No. 22, Public Health Service, Centers for Disease Control.
1991c *Preliminary Budget Submission to DHHS. Fiscal Year 1993*. Agency for Health Care Policy and Research, Public Health Service. Volumes V and VIII.

U.S. Preventive Services Task Force (USPSTF)
1989 *Guide to Clinical Preventive Services: An Assessment of the Effectiveness of 169 Interventions*. Baltimore, MD: Williams & Wilkins.

Wachter, Kenneth W., and M.L. Straf, eds.
1990 *The Future of Meta-Analysis*. Committee on National Statistics, Commission on Behavioral and Social Sciences and Education, National Research Council. New York: Russell Sage Foundation.

Waldo, D.R., S.T. Sonnefeld, D.R. McKusick, et al.
1989 Health Expenditures by Age Group, 1977 and 1987. *Health Care Financing Review* 10(4):111-120.

Walker, A.J.
1990 Results of the Medicare Beneficiary and Physician Focus Groups. Pp. 35-90 in K.N. Lohr, ed., *Medicare: A Strategy for Quality Assurance. Volume II. Sources and Methods*. Washington, DC: National Academy Press.

Ware, J.E., Jr.
1987 Standards for Validating Health Measures: Definition and Content. *Journal of Chronic Diseases* 40(6):473-480.

Wennberg, J.
1990a What is Outcomes Research? Pp. 33-46 in A.C. Gelijns, ed., *Medical Innovation at the Crossroads. Vol. 1. Modern Methods of Clinical Investigation*. Institute of Medicine. Washington, DC: National Academy Press.
1990b Outcomes Research, Cost Containment, and the Fear of Health Care Rationing. *New England Journal of Medicine* 323:1202-1204.

Wennberg, J.E., N.P. Roos, L. Sola, et al.
1987 Use of Claims Data Systems to Evaluate Health Care Outcomes: Mortality and Reoperation Following Prostatectomy. *Journal of the American Medical Association* 257:933-936.

Williams, A.P., W.B. Schwartz, J.P. Newhouse, and B.W. Bennett
1983 How Many Miles to the Doctor? *New England Journal of Medicine* 309:958-963.

Woolhandler, S., and D.U. Himmelstein
- 1989 A National Health Program: A Northern Light at the End of the Tunnel. *Journal of the American Medical Association* 262:2136-2137.
- 1991 Special Article. The Deteriorating Administrative Efficiency of the U.S. Health Care System. *New England Journal of Medicine* 324:1253-1258.

Wunderlich, Gooloo S.
- 1988 Federal Health Statistical System. Unpublished report prepared for the Office of International Health, Office of the Assistant Secretary for Health, Public Health Service, U.S. Department of Health and Human Services, Rockville, MD.